The Johns Hopkins Hospital
1997 Guide to

MEDICAL CARE of PATIENTS WITH HIV INFECTION

Seventh Edition

The Johns Hopkins Hospital 1997 Guide to MEDICAL CARE of PATIENTS WITH HIV INFECTION

Seventh Edition

John G. Bartlett, M.D.

Professor of Medicine
Chief, Division of Infectious Diseases
Johns Hopkins University School of Medicine
Baltimore, Maryland

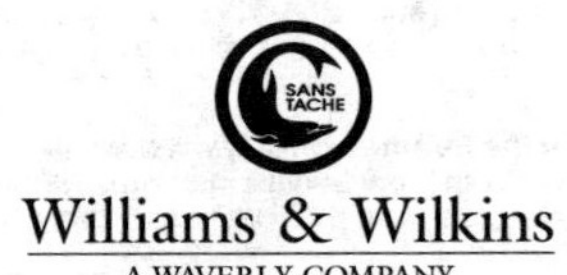

Williams & Wilkins
A WAVERLY COMPANY

BALTIMORE • PHILADELPHIA • LONDON • PARIS • BANGKOK
BUENOS AIRES • HONG KONG • MUNICH • SYDNEY • TOKYO • WROCLAW

Editor: Jonathan W. Pine, Jr
Managing Editor: Molly L. Mullen
Production Coordinator: Marette D. Magargle-Smith
Project Editor: Kathy Gilbert
Typesetter: Maryland Composition Co., Inc.
Printer & Binder: Vicks Lithograph & Printing

351 West Camden Street
Baltimore, Maryland 21201-2436 USA

Rose Tree Corporate Center
1400 North Providence Road
Building II, Suite 5025
Media, Pennsylvania 19063-2043 USA

Accurate indications, adverse reactions, and dosages schedules for drugs are provided in this book, but it is possible that they may change. The reader is urged to review the package information data of the manufacturers of the medications mentioned.

Printed in the United States of America

First Edition 1991
Second Edition 1992
Third Edition 1993
Fourth Edition 1994
Fifth Edition 1995
Sixth Edition 1996

Library of Congress Cataloging-in-Publication Data
Bartlett, John G.
The Johns Hopkins Hospital 1997 guide to the medical care of patients with HIV infection / John G. Bartlett.—7th ed.
p. cm.
Includes bibliographical references and index.
ISBN 0-683-30356-2
1. AIDS (Disease)—Patients—Hospital care. I. Johns Hopkins AIDS Clinic. II. Title.
[DNLM: 1. HIV Infections—therapy. 2. Clinical Protocols—standards. WC 503.2 B289j 1997]
RC607.A26B378 1997
616.97'92—dc21
DNLM/DLC
for Library of Congress 97-16573
CIP

The publishers have made every effort to trace the copyright holders for borrowed material. If they have inadvertently overlooked any, they will be pleased to make the necessary arrangements at the first opportunity.

To purchase additional copies of this book, call our customer service department at **(800) 638-0672** or fax orders to **(800) 447-8438.** For other book services, including chapter reprints and large quantity sales, ask for the Special Sales department.

Canadian customes should call **(800) 268-4178,** or fax **(905) 470-6780.** For all other calls originating outside of the United States, please call **(410) 528-4223** or fax us at **(410) 528-8550.**

Visit Williams & Wilkins on the Internet: **http://www.wwilkins.com** or contact our customer service department at **custserv@wwilkins.com.** Williams & Wilkins customer service representatives are available from 8:30 am to 6:00 pm, EST, Monday through Friday, for telephone access.

98 99 01
2 3 4 5 6 7 8 9 10

PREFACE

The purpose of this document is to provide guidelines for the care of patients with HIV infection. These recommendations reflect the policies of the AIDS Care Program at Johns Hopkins Hospital, where approximately 2,000 patients with this infection are being followed. Recommendations for HIV care change frequently, so the care provider is cautioned that this guideline is dated May 1997.

LIST OF TABLES AND FIGURES

TABLES

FIGURES

CONTENTS

1—HIV Serology and Epidemiology

Indications

Recommendations for persons who should have HIV serologic tests are summarized in Table 1, which is adapted from the recommendations of the CDC (MMWR 1987;36:509; MMWR 1993;42, RR-2). Rapidly evolving improvements in medical care provide the incentive for increased serologic testing. The CDC suggests that hospitals in which seroprevalence rates exceed 1% or in which the case rate of AIDS exceeds 1/1000 discharges should offer serology as a routine admission laboratory test to persons aged 15–54 years (N Engl J Med 1992;327:445; MMWR 1993;42, RR-2). Persons in high-risk categories are also an obvious priority (Table 2).

Informed Consent

The test is considered invasive because of the enormous potential consequences, especially with discrimination in insurance, employment, health care, and personal relationships. Testing should be voluntary with appropriate counseling before and after informed consent. Informed consent is required by law in 41 states, and some laboratories have policies that require the signature of the patient or the legal representative as a contingency for processing. An exception is that many states permit testing of the source with exposures to health care workers. Some areas offer anonymous testing in which all patient identifiers are removed. The usual charge for the test is $30–60; most state and local health departments offer HIV serology at no charge.

Accuracy

Test results are reported as positive, negative, or indeterminate. The standard serologic test requires a positive enzyme-linked immunoabsorbent assay (ELISA) as a screening test and a positive Western blot for confirmation. The usual criteria by Western blot are two of the following: p24, gp41, and gp120/160. Variations in diagnostic criteria and weak bands sometimes cause inconsistencies in reports, but this is unusual. CDC testing of 1400 clinical labs in 1990 showed sensitivity of 99.3% and

Table 1. Recommendations for HIV Serologic Testing

"Guidelines are based on public health considerations for HIV testing, including the principles of counseling before and after testing, confidentiality of personal information, and understanding that a person may decline to be tested without being denied health care or other services except where testing is required by law." Specific recommendations (in no order):

1. Persons who have sexually transmitted diseases
2. High-risk categories: IV drug users, gay and bisexual men, hemophiliacs, regular sexual partners of persons in these categories and persons with known HIV infection; lower incidence risk categories include prostitutes and persons who received transfusions or artificial insemination during 1978–1985
3. Persons who consider themselves at risk or request the test
4. Women at risk who are of child-bearing age. Risk categories are IV drug use; prostitution; male sexual partners who are IV drug users, bisexual, or HIV infected; living in communities or born in countries with high prevalence in women; and blood transfusion between 1978 and 1985
5. All pregnant women (MMWR 44 R-7:1, 1995)
6. Medical evaluation (diagnostic test) for patients with clinical or laboratory findings suggesting HIV infection, including generalized lymphadenopathy; unexplained dementia; chronic, unexplained fever or diarrhea; unexplained weight loss; or diseases that commonly complicate HIV such as chronic or generalized herpes, thrush, oral hairy leukoplakia, other opportunistic infections suggesting unexplained defective cell-mediated immunity,[b] "opportunistic" tumors, including Kaposi's sarcoma and B cell lymphoma, especially if extranodal and aggressive; unexplained cytopenias[b] (anemia, leukopenia, lymphopenia, thrombocytopenia), and unexplained neurologic syndromes[a] (Guillain-Barré syndrome, aseptic meningitis, peripheral neuropathies)
7. Patients with active tuberculosis
8. Recipient and health care workers who are the source of blood or body fluid exposures; body fluids besides blood considered at risk include semen, vaginal secretions, cerebrospinal fluid, synovial fluid, pleural fluid, peritoneal fluid, pericardial fluid, and amniotic fluid, although all occupationally acquired infections in heath care workers have involved blood, bloody body fluids, HIV viral cultures, or SIV in primate workers; body fluids not considered at risk are feces, nasal secretions, sputum, saliva, sweat, tears, urine, and vomitus unless they contain visible blood (MMWR 37:377, 1988). Note: All transmissions of HIV in health care workers have involved blood, bloody body fluids, or viral cultures
9. Health care workers who perform exposure-prone invasive procedures (MMWR 40, RR-8:1, 1991)
10. Hospital admissions for patients aged 15–54 years in facilities where the seroprevalence rate is ≥1% or AIDS case rates are ≥1/1000 discharges (N Engl J Med 327:445, 1992)
11. Donors of blood, semen, and organs (this is the only category in which testing is mandatory in all states)

Adapted from MMWR 36:509, 1987; MMW 40 RR-7:1, 1991, MMWR 42 RR-2, 1993.
[a] Added by author.

Table 2. Seroprevalence of HIV in the United States

Category	Reference	Rate	Comment
Gay men	Am J Epidemiol 126:568, 1987 J AIDS 2:77, 1989 Science 253:37, 1991 JAMA 272:149, 1994 J AIDS 9:514, 1995	14–50%	• Average in Multicenter AIDS Cohort Study (5000 participants) was 36% at entry with 0.5–1.0% annual seroconversion rate; higher in young gay men • Gay men accounted for 41% of the 71,704 newly reported cases of AIDS reported in FY 96
IV drug abusers	JAMA 261:2677, 1989 J AIDS 6:1049, 1993 AIDS 8:263, 1994 Arch Intern Med 155:1305, 1995	1–60%	• Review of 92 studies showed great variation by location: NYC 34–61%; New Jersey 17–29%; Boston 28%; Puerto Rico 45–59%; Detroit 8–12%; San Francisco 5–16%; Miami 5%; New Orleans 1%; Atlanta 10%; Denver 1–5%; Los Angeles 2–5%; Minn: 1% • Annual seroconversion rate: Baltimore 4%; LA nil; Philadelphia 3–15% • IDU accounted for 26% of the 71,704 newly reported cases of AIDS in FY 96
Methadone clinic clients	N Engl J Med 326:375, 1992	1–30%	• Eight city surveys with rates ranging from 0.7% (Seattle) to 28.6% (Newark); average is 9%
Hemophilia	JAMA 253:3409, 1985 J AIDS 7:279, 1994	Type A, 70% Type B, 35%	• Applies to hemophiliacs who received clotting factors before 1985 • Hemophilia accounted for 610 of 71,704 (1%) newly reported AIDS cases in FY 96
Regular sex partners of HIV-infected persons	Arch Intern Med 149:645, 1989 Am J Med 85:472, 1988 JAMA 266:1664, 1991 J AIDS 6:497, 1993 Science 270:1374, 1995	0–58%	• Average is 20–25% for wives of hemophiliac men with HIV infection • Discordant couple study shows efficiency of transmission substantially greater for male N female transmission; annual seroconversion rate for male N female in discordant couples is 3.6% and inversely correlated with condom use • Heterosexual transmission accounted for 12% of 71,704 newly reported cases of AIDS in FY 96
Women (Age 18–59 yrs)	Science 270:1374, 1995	0.15%	• Women accounted for 13,996 of 71,704 (19%) newly reported cases of AIDS in FY 96. This compares to 534 of 8,153 (7%) in 1985. Risk factors in FY 96 reporting: IDU—36%, heterosexual contact—36%; no defined risk—22% • The estimated prevalence of HIV in women aged 18–59 years in the U.S. is 0.15% compared to 0.78% for men

Table 2. *(continued)*

Prostitutes	MMWR 36:157, 1987 JAMA 263:60, 1990	0–57%	• Great variation by location and confounding variable of IVDU: Newark 57%; Washington DC 50%; Miami 19%; San Francisco 6%; Los Angeles 4%; Atlanta 1%; Las Vegas 0
Hospital admissions	N Engl J Med 327:445, 1992	0.2–14.2%	• Average was 4.7% in 20 hospital survey in 1989; 32% of seropositive patients had symptomatic HIV infection or AIDS
College students	N Engl J Med 323:1538, 1990	0.2%	
Child-bearing women and perinatal transmission	JAMA 265:1704, 1991 JAMA 274:952, 1995	0.15%	• Highest rates of HIV in pregnant woman were NYC 0.58%; Washington DC 0.55%; New Jersey 0.49%; Florida 0.45%
Pediatrics	MMWR 45:1005, 1996	0.02%	• Perinatal transmission accounted for 6586 of 548,102 (1.2%) cases of AIDS reported through June, 1996 and 655 of 72,416 (0.9%) of newly reported cases of AIDS reported in FY 96 • The number of perinatally acquired HIV infections decreased from 905 in 1992 to 663 in 1995—a 27% decline
STD clinic clients	STD 19:235, 1992 J AIDS 9:514, 1995 N Engl J Med 326:375, 1992	0.5–11%	• Summary of 552,665 serologic tests in 80 STD clinics from 1988–92 showed HIV seroprevalence was 33% in gay men, 3% in heterosexual men, 2% in heterosexual women and 10% in heterosexual injection drug users
Applicants to military	MMWR 37:67, 1988 J AIDS 3:1168, 1990 J AIDS 10:177, 1995 JAMA 265:1709, 1991	0.13%	• Annual seroconversion rate is 0.02–.03%/yr
Blood donors	N Engl J Med 333:721, 1995	0.02%	• Estimated 18–27 transmission/yr with blood transfusions in the U.S. • Risk is 1 per 450,000–660,000 donations
General population	Science 253:37, 1991 MMWR 30, RR-16, 1990 Science 270:1374, 1995	0.4%	• Annual seroconversion rate based on assumption of 60,000 new infections/year is 0.02% • Seroprevalence in young adult men is estimated at 0.78%

specificity of 99.7% (MMWR 1990;39:380). The rate of false-positive tests in a low-prevalence population with both ELISA and Western blot is about 1/135,000 or 0.0007% (N Engl J Med 1988; 319:961; N Engl J Med 1993;328:1281). The frequency of false-negative results in a high-prevalence population (IV drug abusers with a seroprevalence rate of 30%) is about 0.3% (J Infect Dis 1993;168:327), and in a low-prevalence population (blood donors) it is about 0.001% (N Engl J Med 1991;325:1, 593). The usual cause of false-negative tests is testing during the time between transmission and seroconversion, a period that rarely lasts more than 3 months (N Engl J Med 1991;325:1250; J Infect Dis 1991;164:962, 965). Other causes of false-negative results are agammaglobulinemia or infection with strains that are antigenically distinctive (Lancet 1996;348:176) such as HIV-2 (JAMA 1992;267:2775; Ann Intern Med 1993;118:211) or the subtype O of HIV-1 (Lancet 1993;343:1393; MMWR 1996;45:561; Lancet 1994; 344:1333). HIV-2 has been reported in about 60 patients in the U.S., most of whom have immigrated from or acquired disease in West Africa (MMWR 1995;44:603). Most EIA screening assays used in the U.S. now include antigens to both HIV-1 and HIV-2. There has been only a single case of HIV infection involving subtype O in the U.S. through 7/96 (MMWR 1996;45:561). There is a single case report of a patient with persistently negative serology, AIDS, and positive p24 antigen (MMWR 45:181, 1996).

This experience indicates HIV serology is among the most accurate tests in medicine. Nevertheless, we recommend repeat testing in persons who have positive results with no likely risk factors and those who report positive results without documentation such as those tested with home tests or at an anonymous test site. There is a concern regarding misunderstood results or factitious reporting (Ann Intern Med 1994;121:763). There is no need to confirm test results in patients who have positive results with quantitative HIV RNA assays.

Periodic tests are suggested for patients with negative results who continue to practice high-risk behavior. The frequency is arbitrary, but testing at 6- to 12-month intervals is usually suggested. Annual seroconversion rates in the general population are estimated to be 0.02%, producing an estimated 40,000–80,000 new cases of HIV infection annually in the U.S. (Science 1995; 270:1374). The annual seroconversion rate for gay men is about

0.5–2.0% (higher for young gay men), for IV drug users in geographic areas with a high seroprevalence it is 2–15%, and for discordant couples the rate averages 3.5%/yr depending on regularity of condom use (J AIDS 1993;6:497; J AIDS 1993;6:1049; Am J Epidemiol 1991;134:1175; Arch Intern Med 1995;155:1305).

The most common cause of indeterminate results is a positive ELISA and a single band (usually p24) on a Western blot. This may reflect seroconversion in process, so the test should be repeated in 3–4 months. Persons in low-risk categories with indeterminate test results are virtually never infected with either HIV-1 or HIV-2; repeat testing is likely to show persistence of indeterminant results, and the cause of this pattern is usually not known (N Engl J Med 322:217, 1990). In view of the unnecessary anxiety evoked by knowledge of possible HIV infection, low-risk patients with indeterminate tests should be reassured that HIV infection is very unlikely, but the follow-up test is necessary to provide 100% assurance. When a non–antibody-dependent assay is necessary to confirm or clarify serologic assays, the preferred test is qualitative HIV DNA PCR; this shows sensitivity of 97–98% and specificity of 98% (Ann Intern Med 1996;124: 803).

Alternative Diagnostic Methods to Detect HIV

Alternative tests have been developed to increase access to testing (home test), to improve acceptability of testing (urine or salivary assays), and to reduce the time delay in availability of results.

Home Tests. FDA-approved home tests are as follows:

1. Confide HIV Testing Service (Direct Access Diagnostics; 800-THE TEST)
2. Home Access Express Test (Home Access Health Corp, Hoffman Estates, Ill; 800-HIV-TEST)

These tests are available in pharmacies at $35–50/test. Blood is obtained by lancet, one drop is placed on a filter strip, and this is mailed using an anonymous code for patient identity. Both tests use a double EIA screening test and a confirming test. The consumer telephones for counseling and results in ≥1 wk. Initial studies comparing home tests (Confide) with standard serology show 100% sensitivity and 100% specificity (Arch Intern Med

1997;157:309). The advantage of this method is access to testing by some persons who are reluctant to use standard health care facilities. The main disadvantage is the expense and concern for psychological reactions to results in a non–medical care environment.

Non–Blood Requiring Assays for Physician Use. FDA-approved assays are as follows:

1. Salivary test: OraSure (Epitope Co, Beaverton, OR; 888-ORA-SURE, ext 320). This uses a cotton pad to obtain saliva, which is placed in a vial and submitted to a lab for EIA and Western blot. A study of 3570 persons showed correct results compared with standard serology in 672 of 673 (99.9%) seropositives and 2893 of 2897 (99%) of seronegatives (JAMA 1997; 277:254). Results are available in 3 days by phone or FAX. The cost is $99/three test kits.
2. Urine test: Calypte HIV-1 Urine EIA (Seradyn Inc, 800-428-4007). This test uses urine for EIA screening or dot blot assay (Genie HIV-1/HIV-2, Genetic Systems) (Eur J Clin Microbiol Infect Dis 1996;15:810). Positive results require confirmation by standard serology. The test is supplied as a 192 test kit for $816 or a 480-test kit for $1920; this translates to $4/test.

Rapid Tests. Three FDA approved rapid tests are as follows:

1. SUDS (Murex, Norcross, GA)
2. Recombigen latex agglutination assay (Cambridge Biotech)
3. Genie HIV-1 (Genetic Systems, Seattle, WA)

These tests are analogous to EIA screening, indicating good sensitivity and reduced specificity. The experience with the SUDS test in 6200 patients showed a sensitivity of 99.9–100% and specificity of 98.9–100% (J AIDS 1993;6:115; Am J Emerg Med 1991;9:416; Ann Intern Med 1996;125:471). The cost for SUDS is $283 for 30 assays or $9/test. The advantage is that results are available in 10 minutes. Settings in which rapid screening results are highly desired are for (1) occupational exposures to health care workers and (2) clinical settings where immediate results are desired for patient counseling, especially when reliable follow-up is unlikely; examples are emergency rooms and STD clinics (Ann Intern Med 1996;125:471). Prior studies show that in many settings up to 40% of patients who receive routine serologic tests never return for results (Ann Intern Med 1996;125:471).

Epidemiology (Table 2)

Current estimates are that the seroprevalence of HIV in the U.S. is 0.3% and 650,000–900,000 are living with HIV infection (JAMA 1996;276:126). The total reported with AIDS (1993 definition) for 1981 through 1996 was 573,800. The number of new cases of AIDS has stabilized at 72,967 and 68,473 new cases for 1995 and 1996, respectively (MMWR 1997;46:166). Risk categories for newly reported AIDS cases for FY 96 were gay men—41%, injection drug use—26%, both gay male and injection drug use—4%, heterosexual transmission—12%, blood transfusion—1%, perinatal transmission—1%, and no reported risk—16%.

The total toll of HIV in the U.S. in 1997 is an estimated 775,000 persons living with HIV, including about 223,000 living with AIDS. The total mortality through 1996 was about 350,000. The total number infected through 1997 is estimated at 1,125,000 (775,000 living with HIV and 350,000 deaths). Of this 1,125,000, the major risk categories are sexual transmission (71% of which 87% is gay men), injection drug use (27%), transfusion (2%), and perinatal transmission (1%). These collectively account for 99.8% of all cases in which a transmission category is determined. Less common forms of transmission include transfusion, estimated at 20–30/year with donor screening; occupational exposure, 51–159 (51 confirmed with seroconversion and 108 possible cases); organ transplantation (including 3 post donor screening in 1985); health care worker to patient, 6 (all from the Florida dentist case); household contact, 8; and artificial insemination, 7 (all prior to donor screening in 1985). The CDC review of 68,234 cases with no reported risk through June 1996 showed 36,604 were reclassified, 24,765 are under review, 11,865 had incomplete investigations (died, lost to follow-up declined interview), and 3,152 were from pattern II countries; this left 893 or 0.16% of all reported cases showing no apparent risk.

2—Classification and Natural History

Classification

The current CDC classification system (Table 3) uses three ranges of CD4 cell counts (>500, 200–499, and <200/mm^3) and a matrix of nine mutually exclusive categories. Category B includes most conditions previously classified as AIDS-related complex.

Natural History

Virologic Events and Immune Defense. HIV infection involves the complex interplay of viral replication and immune defenses. Clinical expression in early-stage disease (acute retroviral syndrome) is similar to other acute viral infections; characteristic features in late-stage disease reflect immune destruction, largely because of loss of CD4 cells, which are critical factors for modulating host defenses.

The sequence of events is the following: HIV is transmitted across the mucocutaneous barrier with extension to regional lymph tissue presumably by dendritic cells (days) → massive viremia with the acute retroviral syndrome accompanied by widespread dissemination and extensive involvement of lymph tissue (weeks) → immune response with partial control ascribed to cytotoxic T-cell response (primarily CD8 cells), humoral response (seroconversion at 6–12 weeks), and cytokines (weeks–months) → persistent HIV replication with relatively constant levels of HIV RNA viremia after the "set point" is established about 6 months after HIV transmission and gradual CD4 cell depletion that averages 50/mm^3/year over a mean of 8–10 years → massive destruction of immune system with susceptibility to opportunistic pathogens and opportunistic tumors when the CD4 cell count reaches <200/mm^3 (N Engl J Med 1993; 328:329) (Figure 1).

Two studies with simultaneous publications and nearly identical results (Nature 1995;373:117 and 223) showed the replication rate in midstage disease (patients with CD4 counts ranging from 18 to 460/mm^3) is 10^8–10^9/day, an average of 680,000,000

Table 3. AIDS Surveillance Case Definition for Adolescents and Adults: 1993 (MMWR 41:1–9, 1992)

	Clinical Categories		
CD4 Cell Categories	A Asymptomatic, PGL, or Acute HIV Infection	B Symptomatic (not A or C)[b]	C[a] AIDS Indicator Condition (1987)
1. >500/mm^3 (≥29%)	A1	B1	C1
2. 200–499/mm^3 (14–28%)	A2	B2	C2
3. <200/mm^3 (<14%)	A3	B3	C3

[a] All patients in categories A3, B3, C1–C3 are reported as AIDS based on prior AIDS-indicator conditions (see below) and/or a CD4 cell count of <200/mm^3. AIDS-indicator conditions include three new entries added to the 1987 case definition (MMWR 36:15, 1987): recurrent bacterial pneumonia, invasive cervical cancer, and pulmonary tuberculosis.

[b] Symptomatic conditions not included in category C that *(a)* are attributed to HIV infection or indicate a defect in cell-mediated immunity or *(b)* are conditions considered to have a clinical course or to require management that is complicated by HIV infection. Examples of B conditions include but are not limited to baciliary angiomatosis; thrush; vulvovaginal candidiasis that is persistent, frequent, or poorly responsive to therapy; cervical dysplasia (moderate or severe); cervical carcinoma in situ; constitutional symptoms such as fever (38.5° C) or diarrhea for >1 month; oral hairy leukoplakia; herpes zoster involving two episodes or >1 dermatome; ITP; listeriosis; PID (especially if complicated by a tubo-ovarian abscess); peripheral neuropathy.

Indicator Conditions in Case Definition of AIDS

Candidiasis of esophagus, trachea, bronchi, or lungs
Cervical cancer, invasive[c,d]
Coccidioidomycosis, extrapulmonary[c]
Cryptococcosis, extrapulmonary
Cryptosporidiosis with diarrhea for >1 mo
Cytomegalovirus of any organ other than liver, spleen, or lymph nodes
Herpes simplex with mucocutaneous ulcer for >1 mo or bronchitis, pneumonitis, esophagitis
Histoplasmosis, extrapulmonary[c]
HIV-associated dementia[a]: disabling cognitive and/or motor dysfunction interfering with occupation or activities of daily living
HIV-associated wasting[c]: involuntary weight loss of >10% of baseline plus chronic diarrhea (≥2 loose stools/day for ≥30 days) or chronic weakness and documented enigmatic fever for ≥30 days
Isosporosis with diarrhea for >1 month[c]
Kaposi's sarcoma in patient younger than 60 (or older than 60[c])
Lymphoma of brain in patient younger than 60 (or older than 60[c])
Lymphoma, non-Hodgkin's of B cell or unknown immunologic phenotype and histology showing small, noncleaved lymphoma or immunoblastic sarcoma
Mycobacterium avium or *M. kansasii*, disseminated
Mycobacterium tuberculosis, disseminated[c]
Mycobacterium tuberculosis, pulmonary[c,d]
Nocardiosis[c]
Pneumocystis carinii pneumonia
Pneumonia, recurrent-bacterial[c,d]
Progressive multifocal leukoencephalopathy
Salmonella septicemia (nontyphoid), recurrent[c]
Strongyloidosis, extraintestinal
Toxoplasmosis of internal organ

[c] Requires positive HIV serology.
[d] Added in the revised case definition 1993.

new virions produced daily. The major target of HIV is CD4 cells, and cell destruction represents the effect of viral clearance by cytotoxic T lymphocytes (CTL) or "killer cells" (Nature 1993; 366:22). Current estimates are that the average healthy adult harbors 10^{12} CD4 cells; approximately 10–25% are infected early in the course of HIV infection, and HIV infection results in destruction of about 10^9/day. These data indicate that 30% of the total body HIV burden turns over daily and 6–7% of the CD4 cells turn over daily.

The course of the infection without therapy averages about 10 years from the time of initial infection to an AIDS-defining diagnosis. In some patients, the rate of CD4 cell loss is rampant with counts of <200/mm^3 within 2 years; at the other extreme are "chronic nonprogressors"—defined as patients with HIV infection for >8 years, CD4 count of >500/mm^3, and no antiviral treatment (Lancet 1993;340:863). These variations in course are incompletely understood, but contributing factors that influence the speed of progression and duration of survival are as follows:

- Defective virus (Lancet 1992;340:863)
- Genetic susceptibility of receptor sites (Nature Med 1996; 2:966)
- Age: Duration of survival is inversely correlated with age (Lancet 1996;347:1573)
- Major histocompatibility genes (Nature Med 1996;4:405)
- Immune response: Primarily T-cell response in early-stage disease (Science 1996;271:324; PNAS 1997;94:254)
- Severity of symptoms with the acute HIV syndrome (BMJ 1989;299:154; JID 1993;168:1490)
- Plasma level of HIV RNA after the set point is established (Science 1996;272:1167)
- Medical interventions. The following interventions are associated with a significant increase in survival:
    1. Antiretroviral therapy (N Engl J Med 1987;317:185; JAMA 1989;262:2045); Ann Intern Med 1995;122:850)
    2. *P. carini* prophylaxis (JAMA 1988;259:118)
    3. *M. avium* prophylaxis (N Engl J Med 1996;335:384)
    4. Care by a physician with HIV experience (NEJM 1996; 334:701)

Viral transmission. Risk categories for 72,416 newly reported AIDS cases in FY 96 were: gay men—41%, injection drug

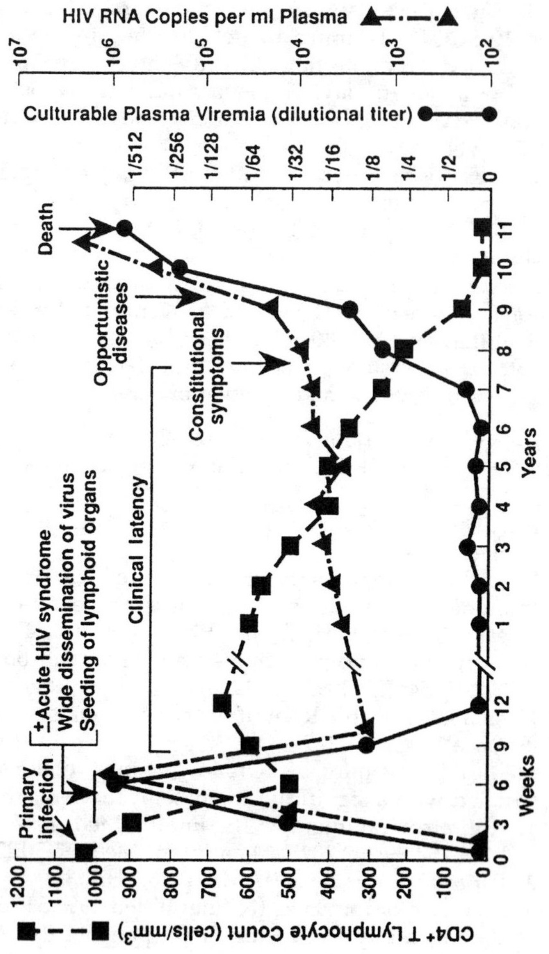
HIV RNA Copies per ml Plasma
10^7
10^6
10^5
10^4
10^3
10^2
Culturable Plasma Viremia (dilutional titer)
1/512
1/256
1/128
1/64
1/32
1/16
1/8
1/4
1/2
0
Death
Opportunistic diseases
Constitutional symptoms
Clinical latency
±Acute HIV syndrome
Wide dissemination of virus
Seeding of lymphoid organs
Primary infection
CD4+ T Lymphocyte Count (cells/mm3)
1200
1100
1000
900
800
700
600
500
400
300
200
100
0
0
3
6
9
12
Weeks
1
2
3
4
5
6
7
8
9
10
11
Years

Figure 1. The typical course of HIV infection without therapy. The initial event is the acute retroviral syndrome accompanied by a decline in CD4 cell count (*closed squares*), high-level cultivable HIV plasma viremia (*closed circles*), and high plasma concentrations of HIV RNA (*closed triangles*). Clinical symptoms usually resolve spontaneously in 1–3 weeks; this recovery is accompanied by a rapid decline in plasma viremia, reflecting CTL response (Science 1996;272:505). The CD4 cell count may return toward baseline, although some studies show no rebound (Ann Intern Med 1996;125:257), and then shows a linear decline that averages $50/mm^3$/year. The subsequent course generally shows a prolonged period of clinical latency that is accompanied by high rates of HIV replication with an average of approximately 10^9 new virions/day. Concentrations of HIV RNA predict the course (about 10^3/mL for slow-progressors, and $>10^5$/mL for rapid progressors). The CD4 cell count decline (CD4 slope) is often accelerated during late-stage disease as indicated by the "inflection point" of the CD4 slope, and this is accompanied by increased levels of HIV RNA. A CD4 cell count of $200/mm^3$ is generally regarded as the threshold at which patients become vulnerable to opportunistic infections. The median time to an AIDS-defining complication after reaching $200/mm^3$ is 18–24 months, the median survival after a CD4 count of $200/mm^3$ is 3.1 years, and the median survival after an AIDS-defining complication is 1.3 years. (This is without antiretroviral therapy.) With no therapy directed against HIV and no PCP prophylaxis, the average time from viral transmission to an AIDS-defining diagnosis is about 10 years, Data provided for the CD4 cell count decline are averages based on natural history studies in MACs (J Infect Dis 1993;168:149; J AIDS 1995;8:66). There is substantial individual variation; some patients have a rapid decline in CD4 cell counts after acute retroviral syndrome, and 5–15% are considered chronic nonprogressors with CD4 cell counts exceeding $500/mm^3$ for more than 8 years (J AIDS 1995;8:496). Given comparable care, there is no significant difference in rates of progression based on sex, race, or risk category. Variations in rates of progression in untreated adults reflect both viral factors (virulence) and host defense, especially CTL response (Science 1996;271:324; PNAS 1997;94:254). (From Fauci A et al. Ann Intern Med 1996;124:654.)

use—26%, both gay male and IDU—4%, heterosexual transmission—12%, blood transfusion—1%, perinatal transmission—1%, and no reported risk category—16%. The efficiency of transmission depends on the type of exposure and viral load of the infected source. The estimate with unprotected sexual contact in which one partner is infected is 0.2% (1/500) (STD 1997;24:102); it is higher during the acute retroviral syndrome and late-stage disease when the level of plasma viremia is much higher: the efficiency of transmission is 3- to 7-fold higher with STDs associated with an inflammatory reaction or genital ulcer, and it is up to 20 times more efficiently transmitted from male to female (J AIDS 1993;6:497; JAMA 1991;266:1664). The frequency and concentration of HIV in urethral specimens increases with urethritis and decreased CD4 counts (JID 1995;172:1469) and in vaginal secretions with vaginal discharge, cervical mucopus, or low CD4 count (JID 1997;175:57).

Acute HIV infection. This illness generally occurs 1–3 weeks after an exposure such as a needle-stick injury in a health care worker or sexual exposure (Ann Intern Med 1996;125:257; Ann Intern Med 1993;118:913; JID 1994;168:1490). The frequency with which this syndrome is observed in patients who have sequential blood samplings documenting seroconversion is 50–90% (BMJ 1989;299:154). Clinical features (Table 4) are those

Table 4. Acute HIV Infection

Symptomatic disease: 50–89%
Frequency of correct diagnosis with medical consultation: 25%
Incubation period (HIV exposure to onset of symptoms): 2–6 wk
Symptoms and signs

Fever	96%	Diarrhea	32%
Adenopathy	74%	Nausea or vomiting	27%
Pharyngitis	70%	Hepatosplenomegaly	14%
Rash	70%	Thrush	12%
Myalgias	54%	Meningoencephalitis	6%
Headache	32%	Peripheral neuropathy	6%

Duration of symptoms (mean): 1–2 wk
Laboratory tests: p24 antigenemia (1200–4200 pg/mL), plasma viremia with high titer (peak of 10^5–10^7 copies per mL), high-titer HIV-1 in peripheral blood mononuclear cells (10^2–10^4 tissue culture infective doses per mL), HIV-1 serologic test negative or indeterminant.

Adapted from Niu MT et al. JID 1993;168:1490 and Schacker T et al. Ann Intern Med 1996; 125:257.

of an infectious mononucleosis-like illness with fever, adenopathy, hepatosplenomegaly, sore throat, myalgias, morbilliform rash, mucocutaneous ulceration, diarrhea, and leukopenia with atypical lymphocytes (Ann Intern Med 1993;118:913; JID 1994; 168:1490; Ann Intern Med 1996;125:257). Some patients have neurologic symptoms such as aseptic meningitis, Guillain-Barré syndrome, or acute psychosis. The five most common clinical features in the Seattle study were fever (mean of 38.9° C), sore throat, fatigue, malaise, and weight loss (average 5 kg); 17% were hospitalized and 24% had signs of aseptic meningitis (Ann Intern Med 1996;125:257). The febrile illness is self-limited, usually lasting 1–3 weeks. Laboratory studies show high concentrations of HIV in the blood as indicated by quantitative virology or p24 antigen assays accompanied by negative or indeterminate serologic tests for antibody. The most sensitive tests for antigen detection are quantitative or qualitative HIV RNA (Transfusion 1994;34:376). There is also a decrease in CD4 cell counts, sometimes to levels associated with major opportunistic infections such as PCP (Lancet 1993;342:24). A placebo-controlled trial showed AZT treatment in this early stage of infection was associated with a delay in the onset of opportunistic infections and an increase in CD4 cell counts at 6 months; long-term benefits are unknown (N Engl J Med 1995;333:401; also see JID 1997;175: 1051).

Seroconversion. Seroconversion generally takes place 6–12 weeks after transmission (N Engl J Med 1991;325:1250; J Infect Dis 1991;164:962, 965; Epidemiol Rev 1993;15:503; Lancet 1989; 2:637). The CTL response precedes humoral response and is accompanied by a sharp reduction in plasma concentrations of HIV RNA copies (PNAS 1997;94:254) and resolution of symptoms of acute HIV infection.

Early HIV disease. This represents the period between seroconversion to 6 months following HIV transmission. During this time there is substantial variation in plasma concentrations of HIV RNA and CD4 counts. At about 6 months the plasma levels of HIV RNA are established at a set point that shows minimal variation over several years in the absence of antigenic stimuli (intercurrent illness or immunizations) or antiretroviral therapy (Ann Intern Med 1996;125:257). This set point dictates the subsequent rate of progression: high concentrations

(>100,000 copies/mL) are associated with a CD4 slope of −76 cells/mm^3/year and a median survival of 4.4 years; low concentrations (<5,000 copies/mL) are associated with a CD4 slope of −36 cells/mm^3/year and a median survival exceeding 10 years (Mellors J, et al. Ann Intern Med, in press).

Symptomatic HIV infection. Complications of HIV infection are ascribed to direct effects of the virus and to the consequences of immunosuppression:

- Direct effect of HIV: Acute HIV syndrome, persistant generalized lymphadenopathy (PGL), HIV-associated dementia, lymphocytic interstitial pneumonia (LIP), HIV-associated nephropathy, and progressive immunosuppression. Other possible consequences are anemia, neutropenia, thrombocytopenia, cardiomyopathy, myopathy, peripheral neuropathy, chronic meningitis, polymyositis, and Guillain-Barre syndrome.
- Immunosuppression results in opportunistic infections and tumors, primarily reflecting compromised cell-mediated immunity.

The correlation between these complications and the CD4 count as a barometer of immunocompetence is summarized in Table 5. In each instance the CD4 strata assigned is the highest in which the designated complication is likely to be encountered; virtually all conditions increase in frequency with progressive decline in CD4 count.

Early complications generally represent complications of HIV infection per se or they are infections involving relatively virulent microbes that do not require severe immunosuppression for clinical expression. The latter include vaginal candidiasis, pneumococal pneumonia, tuberculosis, and zoster. The complications designated as AIDS-defining (Table 5) generally occur with severe immunosuppression to CD4 counts below 200/mm^3 and usually below 100/mm^3. The relative frequency of these complications as the original AIDS-defining diagnosis is summarized in Table 6 and their frequency as a cause of death is summarized in Table 7.

Asymptomatic infection. During this period the patient is asymptomatic or may have persistent generalized lymphadenopathy. There is usually a gradual decline in the CD4 cell count in untreated patients averaging 40–60/mm^3/year according to

Table 5. Correlation of Complications with CD4 Cell Strata

CD4 Cell Count[a]	Infections	Noninfectious
>500/mm^3	Candida vaginitis	Persistent generalized lymphadenopathy (PGL) Polymyositis Chronic meningitis Guillain-Barre Syndrome
200–500/mm^3	Pneumococcal and other bacterial pneumonia (90)[b] Pulmonary TB (90–180) Kaposi sarcoma (30–130) Herpes zoster (150–170) Thrush Oral hairy leukoplakia	Cervical intraepithelial neoplasia Cervical cancer (180) Myopathy Anemia Idiopathic thrombocytopenic purpura
<200/mm^3	*P. carinii* pneumonia (40–120) Candida esophagitis (30–80) Disseminated/chronic Herpes simplex (40–110) Toxoplasmopsis (20–40) Cryptococcosis (20–60) Disseminated histoplasmosis (30) Disseminated coccidioidomycosis (40) Cryptosporidiosis, chronic (40–130) Progressive multifocal leukoencephalopathy (PML) (40–110) Microsporidiosis (<100) Miliary/extrapulmonary TB (40)	Wasting (20–100) B-cell lymphoma (30–60) Cardiomyopathy (25) Peripheral neuropathy HIV-associated dementia (20–60) CNS lymphoma (20) Cardiomyopathy HIV-associated nephropathy
<50/mm^3	CMV disease (10–20) Disseminated *M. avium* complex (10–20)	

[a] Indicated complications occur with increased frequency at lower CD4 strata; lymphomas may occur at any CD4 cell strata, but are most frequent with counts <200/mm^3.

[b] No. in ( ) indicates the approximate median CD4 cell count at the time of the diagnosis (See CID 1995;21 (Suppl 1):56; JAMA 1992;267:1798; Ann Intern Med 1996;124:633). Some values are ranges indicating multiple sources: (CDC, MACS (A. Munoz, personal communication)).

Table 6. Frequency of Initial AIDS-Defining Diagnosis

	Initial AIDS Defining Diagnosis[a]		Frequency (%) among All Patients[b]
	1990 (%)	1995 (%)	
Pneumocystis pneumonia	49	28	75–85
HIV wasting syndrome	17	14	70–90
Candida esophagitis	13	11	20–30
Kaposi's sarcoma	11	6	15–25
HIV-associated dementia	6	4	40 70
Disseminated CMV	6	6	80–90
Toxoplasmosis encephalitis	5	3	5–15
Disseminated *M. avium* infection	4	4	30–40
Lymphoma	3	2	3–5
Chronic mucocutaneous herpes simplex	3	4	10–25
Cryptococcal meningitis	3	4	8–12
Cryptosporidiosis	2	2	5–10
Tuberculosis	—	5[c]	4–20

[a] Frequency according to CDC criteria for AIDS 1987–1992 as reported for newly diagnosed cases in 1990 and for 1995.
[b] Estimated lifetime frequency among all patients with AIDS without prophylaxis.
[c] Added in the revised case definition of 1993.

sequential assays in large cohorts of patients followed for prolonged periods (J Infect Dis 1992;165:352). This decline is not linear in an individual owing to biologic variations in the individual patient and substantial variations based on laboratory technology (Clin Infect Dis 1995;21:1121). As noted above, some patients have a rapid decline in CD4 cells (rapid progressors),

Table 7. Causes of Death in U.S. Patients Dying of AIDS

	1987 n = 10,001	1992 n = 24,230
Pneumonia-unspecified cause	18%	18%
P. carinii pneumonia	33%	14%
Non-TB mycobacteria	7%	12%
Bacterial septicemia	9%	12%
Kaposi sarcoma	12%	10%
CMV disease	5%	10%
Non-Hodgkins lymphoma	4%	6%
Toxoplasmosis	5%	5%
Cryptococcosis	8%	5%
Tuberculosis	3%	4%
PML	1%	2%

Based on ICD-9 codes for cause of death (CDC, Ann Intern Med 1995;123:933).

and some have sustained counts >500/mm^3 for 8 years (chronic nonprogressors). The lower limit for the normal range for CD4 counts in most labs is 400–450/mm^3. These levels in HIV infected patients indicate substantial loss of immune function, although clinical expression with opportunistic infection is unusual with CD4 counts >200/mm^3 and the first AIDS-defining OI occurs with an average CD4 count of 70/mm^3 (Am J Epidemiol 1995; 141:645).

3—Diagnostic Evaluation

Summary of Guidelines of U.S. Public Health Service—Infectious Diseases Society of America (CID 1995;21:S1:)

Initial Evaluation

1. Obtain a *complete medical history* with emphasis on OIs including constitutional symptom, candidiasis, pneumonia, gastrointestinal symptoms, results of PPD, date of last PPD, treatment of TB, STDs, Pap smear results, date of last Pap smear.
2. Determine *HIV risk behavior* and access ongoing high-risk behavior that placed patient contacts at risk and behavior that places patient at risk for OIs.
3. *Patient exam* with emphasis on candidiasis, funduscopic exam, lymphadenopathy, lungs, hepatosplenomegaly, skin disease, STDs, gynecologic exam.
4. *Laboratory tests*

    - HIV serology (confirmed test or positive HIV RNA)
    - CBC
    - CD4 count
    - Plasma quantitative HIV RNA
    - Chemistry profile
    - Toxoplasma serology (IgG)
    - Chest x-ray (The utility of a baseline chest x-ray is question-

able in patients with a negative PPD [Arch Intern Med 1996;156:191])

- PPD (unless history of positive PPD or history of TB treatment)
- CMV serology (if low risk)
- STD screen; RPR or VDRL, ±GC and chlamydia screen (women)
- Hepatitis screen: anti-HBc (to determine candidates for HBV vaccine); HBsAg and anti-HCV (to detect active hepatitis if unexplained elevated transaminase levels)
- Pap smear (if none in past year)

5. *PCP prophylaxis* if reliable history of PCP, thrush, or CD4 count ever known to be $<200/mm^3$
6. *M. avium* prophylaxis if CD4 count ever known to be $<50/mm^3$
7. *Pneumococcal vaccine* if not given in past 5 years. Note: This vaccine should be delayed until the second viral burden test is completed

Counseling

Detailed information regarding medical, psychological, public health, and social implications should be provided to persons with HIV infection. The checklist of items covered in this counseling session used at The Johns Hopkins Hospital is provided in Table 8. Many or most points covered will need to be reiterated at a subsequent visit that is usually scheduled 2 weeks later when the initial laboratory test results are completed and the second baseline viral burden test is obtained. Physicians are cautioned to be sensitive about what may be obvious: HIV infection has historically been viewed as invariably progressive with morbid late consequences that often include dementia, debilitating diarrhea, and emaciation eventuating in what many fear most—death without dignity. The medical tragedy has been compounded by social stigma that has made HIV-infected persons the lepers of the 20th century. The point to emphasize is that these patients desperately need the compassion and sensitivity that characterize the best practitioners of our profession. The recent past has brought new promise in the effectiveness of therapy and public perceptions of the disease have improved;

nevertheless, much of the former lore persists and some patients have unrealistic expectations. Included in the counseling should be the following.

Natural History of HIV Infection. The average time from HIV transmission to serious complications in the absence of treatment is approximately 10 years (J Infect Dis 1988;158:1360; BMJ 1990;301:1183). Nevertheless, there is considerable variation, and some untreated patients have stable CD4 cell counts and remain asymptomatic for 8–10 years or longer (Lancet 1993; 340:863); in the San Francisco cohort of gay men 19% were asymptomatic 11 years after seroconversion, and in the Multicenter AIDS Cohert Study (MACS) it is estimated that 13% will remain asymptomatic without therapy at least 20 years after HIV transmission (J AIDS 1994;8:496). These studies were largely completed before the time in which there could be a substantial impact by treatment strategies that are now considered routine practice. Therapeutic interventions associated with significant prolongation of survival in controlled trials are antiretroviral therapy, *P. carinii* prophylaxis, and *M. avium* prophylaxis. In late 1995 and early 1996, there was the introduction of 3TC, non-nucleoside reverse transcriptase inhibitors and protease inhibitors—drugs that have the most substantial impact on HIV in vivo in terms of quantitative virology and CD4 response; this brought a new wave of enthusiasm for antiretroviral therapy and new hope that these drugs would make it possible for most patients to be "chronic nonprogressors." The patient should be aware that (1) there are extraordinary demands with commonly recommended regimens in terms of toxicity, compliance, and pill burden; (2) there are as yet no cures; (3) studies with the new drugs confirm potent activity in most recipients up to 1–2 years, but there are no studies to confirm longer benefit. Despite those limitations, treatment strategies in current use are likely to delay progression, and this may persist indefinitely or permit access to these new therapeutic options in the future.

Positive serology indicates viral carriage and risk of transmission. Sexual intercourse, needle sharing by drug users, and maternal-fetal transmission account for at least 99.5% of all new HIV infections. Prevention of transmission accordingly includes abstention from intercourse or "safer sex" (condoms), avoidance of sharing needles or works by intravenous drug users,

Table 8. The Johns Hopkins Hospital HIV Post-Test Assessment

Test Results: ELISA ________________ Western Blot ________________
Conclusion ____
Date of Test ________________ Date of Counseling ________________
Requesting Physician ____
Reason for Test ____

	Yes	No
1. Purpose of Test		
a) A positive HIV test (ELISA & Western Blot) indicates infection with the virus that causes AIDS. False positives occasionally occur and are most likely in low-risk groups.	☐	☐
b) A positive ELISA screen and an indeterminant Western blot in a patient without an AIDS diagnosis may represent early infection or a false-positive ELISA screen. A repeat test in 2–3 months is advised.		
2. Prognosis		
About 50% of patients with a positive test will go on to develop AIDS within 10 years after HIV is acquired without treatment. The prognosis for an individual infected with HIV beyond that time is now known; but nearly all will eventually develop AIDS.	☐	☐
3. Transmission	☐	☐
A person with a positive test is considered infectious and is capable of transmitting the infection to others. The infection is usually transmitted through sexual contact and sharing of needles. Infection through other body fluids (saliva, urine, feces) is theoretically possible, but is not known to occur. It is not known that HIV therapy will reduce the probability of transmission with high-risk behavior.		
4. Risk Reduction		
a. Reduce/limit the number of sexual parters.	☐	☐
b. When engaged in sexual contract, do not pass or receive body fluids, particularly blood, semen, and vaginal secretions. Use condoms for all sexual contacts.	☐	☐
c. Do not share needles.	☐	☐
d. Do not donate blood, plasma, body organs, semen, or other body tissue.	☐	☐
e. Do not share items such as razors and toothbrushes.	☐	☐

5. **Sexual/needle partner referral**
   All sexual/needle partners for a minimum of the last year (preferably the last 2 years) should be notified and referred for testing and counseling. ☐ ☐
6. **Medical Evaluation**
   Patients with HIV infection need regular medical care by a physician with appropriate expertise. This has become a critical component of HIV care because of the medical treatments now available that are highly effective in delaying progression. ☐ ☐
   Care Provider ______________
7. **Who Should Be Told**
   When seeking medical or dental care, the patient should inform the care provider of the positive status so that appropriate tests will be done. There is usually no need to tell others. ☐ ☐
8. **Pregnancy**
   A woman with HIV infection should not get pregnant and should use a reliable contraceptive method other than condoms. A women with HIV infection who gives birth has a 20–30% chance of spreading the infection to her child during pregnancy, delivery, or breastfeeding. This risk is reduced to about 8% with AZT treatment. Women with children of preschool or grade school age may consider having their children tested for HIV. ☐ ☐

Patient understanding ______________________________

Special problems ______________________________

Suggested baseline tests for medical evaluation: ______________________________

____

Counselor ______________________________

and avoidance of pregnancy or breastfeeding. New therapies reduce viral burden, but this is not known to be accompanied by reduced efficiency of transmission; thus, standard methods to protect others should apply.

Pregnancy in a seropositive woman carries an 8–25% risk of HIV infection in the infant; the rate is highest for women with high viral RNA concentrations or low CD4 cell counts (Lancet 1992;339:1007; JAMA 1996;275:640). ACTG trial 076 showed the rate of perinatal transmission was reduced with AZT treatment from 25% in the placebo group to 8% in AZT recipients (N Engl J Med 1994;331:1173). Viral transmission may occur in utero, at delivery, or with breastfeeding. It is not currently known if the 8% rate can be further reduced by more aggressive therapy. Condoms are not regarded as adequate for birth control and should be used in conjunction with other methods such as birth control pills. The typical pregnancy failure rate for first year use is 8% for oral contraceptives, 15% for male condoms, and 26% for periodic abstinence; the failure rate with consistent use of oral contraceptives is 0.1% and for consistent use of male condoms is 2% (MMWR 1993;42:491).

Notification. Persons with a need to know that the patient is infected are those placed at risk: sex partners and needle-sharing partners. These people should be informed as a public health concern and to promote testing and early treatment. Physicians and dentists involved in care should also be told. Infected health care workers should notify their employer according to institutional guidelines (MMWR 1991;40, RR-8:1; JAMA 1993; 269:1843). There is no necessity to notify others, e.g., friends, family, employers, coworkers, landlords; the patient should be forewarned of possible harsh repercussions of such disclosure. Health care workers who are aware of persons who are knowingly placed at risk have a duty to warn in the event that the patient refuses to disclose this information.

Psychological response to notification of HIV infection is similar to that found with notification of any lethal disease. Virtually all patients have an adjustment disorder with anxiety, depression, insomnia, somatic concerns, and/or suicidal thoughts. Appropriate support often requires the assistance of a mental health professional, especially if the adjustment disorder is prolonged, if there is a major depression, or if the patient is suicidal. For anxiety, our recommendation is lorazepam (Ativan), 0.5–1.0 mg bid, but this should be given for no longer than 3 days because of dependency potential.

Resources. Resources for patient services, clinical trials, and financial assistance are available from community-based organizations, local academic institutions, and special entitlement programs through regional health departments. Recommended sources of information for patients follow.

PWP Coalition of New York: 50 W 17th St NY, NY; publishes "PWP Coalition Newsletter," a monthly newsletter on alternative medicines and outreach activities: 212-647-1420; AIDS information hot line: 800-828-3280

National HIV and AIDS Hotline: a 24 hr/day hotline contracted by the CDC: 800:342-AIDS; Spanish: 800-344-SIDA

Local AIDS Services: a national directory with a listing of services by geographic location from the U.S. Conference of Mayors, 1620 Eye St N.W., Washington, DC 20006 ($15): 202-293-7330

HIV/AIDS Treatment Information Service: a U.S. Public Health Service free telephone reference service for patients and providers: 1-800-448-0440 or write PO Box 6303, Rockville, MD 20849-6303

Therapeutic Trials Hotline: National Institute of Allergy and Infectious Diseases: 1-800-TRIALS-A

American Foundation for AIDS Research (AmFar): "AIDS/HIV Experimental Treatment Directory" (updated quarterly) and "AIDS Targeted Information Newsletter." 212-682-7440 ($125/year).

Gay Men's Health Crisis (GMHC): "Treatment Issues," GMHC, Department of Medical Information, 129 West 20th Street, New York, NY 10011: 1-212-807-6655 ($30/year; reliable reviews of therapeutics); Dept of Education and Advocacy, 212-337-3505

National AIDS Hotline: contracted through CDC for general information including local services: English (24 hours/day, 7 days/week) 1-800-342-AIDS; Spanish (8:00 a.m.–2:00 p.m. 7 days/week) 1-800-344-SIDA; deaf (10:00 a.m.–10:00 p.m. Mon–Fri) 1-800-243-7889

National AIDS Clearinghouse: a library for information with publications, videos, lists of service, and community-based organizations, P.O. Box 6303, Rockville, MD 20849-6303: 1-800-458-5231

The Guide to Living with HIV Infection: 1997 edition, The Johns Hopkins University Press, 2715 North Charles Street, Baltimore, MD 21218-4319 (paperback $15.95)

Bulletin of Experimental Treatments for AIDS (BETA): San Francisco AIDS Foundation; request from BETA Subscriber Services, Infocom Group, 1250 45th Street, Suite 200, Emoryville, CA 94608-2924: 1-800-959-1059 [$75/year; trial subscription without payment offered (suggested for the sophisticated reader)]

Legal Issues/Civil Rights: Office of Civil Rights, U.S. Department of Health and Human Services, P.O. Box 13716, Mail Stop 07, Philadelphia, PA 19101; 1-215-596-6109 Social Security—disability qualifications: 1-800-772-1213

National Institute on Drug Abuse Hotline: English 1-800-662-4357; Spanish 1-800-662-9832

Project Inform: 1-800-822-7422—Treatment hotline

National Association of People with AIDS: 202-898-0414—Information about local resources, including support groups, mail order pharmacy, update information on new treatments, and 2 publications: "Medical Alert" (treatments) and "Active Voice" (advocacy)

PWA Newsline: 1-800-828-3280—counseling, information on medications, referral for support group, and referrals for services including services for persons outside the U.S.

"Wellness": Exercise, Smoking, Alcohol. Medical care should include appropriate attention to nutrition, exercise, continued work, and other facets of "wellness." Depression does not appear to accelerate disease progression (JAMA 1993;270:2563). Three separate studies have demonstrated deleterious consequences of smoking with increased rates of PCP and more rapid progression to AIDS (AIDS 1990;4:327). It is unknown if effective PCP prophylaxis would nullify the disadvantage. Strenuous exercise as done by Olympic athletes or marathon runners is deleterious to immune function with increased susceptibility to common viral infections, but is not known to reduce cell-mediated immunity; moderate exercise such as jogging or bicycle riding has no apparent adverse effect on immune function and may improve sense of well-being. Alcohol in moderation (1 drink/day) has no adverse health consequences including problems with immune function, infections, rates of liver disease, or rates of hepatitis with AZT, INH, etc.; obviously, alcohol may reduce inhibitions and enhance high-risk behavior and also promote side effects of psychiatric or sedative drugs. Of particular concern is the effect alcohol has on compliance with complex medical regimens, especially binge drinking. Nutrition needs emphasis, but it is unknown whether specific diets, vitamin supplements, or mineral supplements are advantageous (Lancet 338:86, 1991; Nutr Rev 1990;48:393). Unusual diets such as macrobiotic diet and megavitamins may be dangerous. "Traditional therapy" (e.g., PCP prophylaxis, tuberculosis control, and antiretroviral treatment) has become important in prolonged survival.

Prevention of Opportunistic Infection

(Recommendations of U.S. Public Health Service/IDSA Guidelines (MMWR 1995;44:RR-8); Ann Intern Med 1996;124:348)

Pets. The major concern with pets is that they may carry the microbes that cause diarrhea in patients, primarily *Cryptosporidia, Salmonella*, and *Campylobacter*. The following precautions will help avoid this type of exposure: Veterinary consultation should be obtained if the pet develops diarrhea. When obtaining a new pet, avoid animals less than 6 months of age, pets with diarrhea, stray animals, and animals from facilities that have poor hygienic conditions. Wash hands after handling pets and especially before eating and avoid contact with stool. If a pet develops diarrhea, it should be examined by a veterinarian.

Cats are of particular concern due to risk of exposure to toxoplasmosis and Bartonella, as well as the microbes that cause diarrhea. It is best to obtain a cat over 1 year of age, and a cat in good health. Litter boxes should be cleaned daily, preferably by someone who has neither HIV infection nor is pregnant. If this must be done by a HIV-infected person, hands should be washed thoroughly afterward to reduce the risk. Cats should be kept indoors, should not hunt, and should not be fed raw or undercooked meat since all of these increase the risk of toxoplasmosis. Bartonella is transmitted by bites and scratches of cats, and these should be avoided and should be cleaned promptly when they occur. It is not suggested to declaw a cat or test the animal for either toxoplasmosis or Bartonella infection.

With regard to other pets, healthy birds may be the source of cryptococcus or Histoplasma. Reptiles such as snakes and turtles may carry *Salmonella.* Aquariums are generally safe, but gloves should be used for cleaning to reduce exposure to *Mycobacterium marinum.* Nonhuman primates like monkeys should be avoided.

Food. The major risk with food and fluids is exposure to the microbes that cause diarrhea. There are several, but the most important are *Cryptosporidia* and *Salmonella. Salmonella* is often present in eggs and poultry, and undercooked meat is a common source of Toxoplasmosis. The usual recommendation is to avoid raw or undercooked eggs, including the foods that often contain raw eggs such as hollandaise sauce and Caesar salad dressing. Also avoid raw or undercooked poultry, seafood, and meat. Poultry and meat should be cooked until it is no longer pink in the middle. Produce should be washed well before it is eaten. Patients should be reminded of the possibility of exposure to undercooked meats or other products through contact with cutting boards, counters, knives, and hands used in preparation; all should be washed carefully.

Warn patients to not drink directly from lakes or rivers due to the risk of *cryptosporidiosis.* There are sometimes community outbreaks of diarrhea in which there is a "boil-water" advisory. At this time the water should be boiled for 1 minute to remove the risk of *Cryptosporidia* and other disease-causing microbes. Other options are submicron personal-use water filters and/or bottled water. The submicron filter recommended is one that is labeled as "absolute" 1 μm filter; the best are those labeled to show they meet National Sanitation Foundation Standard number 53 for "cyst removal." Note that many filters labeled 1 μm are not standardized and are consequently not recommended. It is not generally recommended that HIV-infected persons boil the water or use tap water filtration if there isn't an advisory, but some may choose to use these precautions to be extra cautious.

Travel. The greatest health risk to persons with and without HIV infection is visits to developing countries, and the major problem is microbes that contaminate food and water. The things to avoid are raw fruits and vegetables, raw or undercooked seafood or meat, tap water, ice made from tap water, nonpasteurized milk and dairy products, and items purchased from street vendors. The preferred foods are those that are steaming hot, fruits that can be peeled by the traveler, bottled water, hot coffee or tea, or anything with alcohol in it. Water may also be treated with iodine or chlorine, but this is not as effective as a rolling boil for 1 minute.

Antibiotics to prevent infections during travel to developing countries are usually not recommended, but they may be for some HIV-infected patients who are considered at high risk. A common recommendation is for a fluoroquinolone. Trimethoprim-sulfamethoxazole is sometimes used, and many travelers may already be taking this to prevent *Pneumocystis* pneumonia. It is important to be aware of the side effects of TMP-SMX when taken for prophylaxis during travel since these may appear like some tropical disease. The most common reaction is a rash and fever, and the only treatment necessary is to simply stop the drug. For travelers to developing countries who do not take antibiotics, it is generally recommended to take two types of medications in the event that diarrhea develops. One drug, like loperamide, is used for the control of mild diarrhea. A fluoroquinolone is taken if the diarrhea is more serious, if it is accompanied by fever, or if there is blood in the stool. These recommendations are generally made on the assumption that most diarrhea in travelers is easily controlled and access to quality health care may be difficult to obtain.

Vaccines are often required or recommended for travel, and recommendations are made in Table 9. The general rule is that HIV-infected persons cannot receive live virus vaccines. If there is anticipated exposure to typhoid fever, the recommendation is for the inactivated injected vaccine rather than the live vaccine form that is given by mouth. For yellow fever, the only vaccine is a live virus vaccine that has uncertain safety in people with HIV infection; if there is travel to an area with yellow fever, it may be necessary to obtain a letter indicating vaccination waiver and there needs to be extra caution in avoiding mosquito bites. Killed vaccines are not a problem, and these include the stan-

Table 9. Vaccines for Travel

Disease	Acceptable	Avoid	Comment
Polio	eIPV	Oral polio	Close contracts should also receive eIPV
Hepatitis A	—	HAV vaccine	Live virus vaccine; use gammaglobulin
Typhoid	Typhim V_1	Ty21a (Vivotif)	Inactivated parenteral vaccine is also acceptable
Jap B enceph.	JBE Vaccine	—	
Yellow fever	—	Vaccine	Advise patient of risk and risk prevention (mosquito), and provide waiver

dard diphtheria-tetanus (Dt), rabies, and Japanese encephalitis vaccines.

Travelers need to be aware about the types of infectious diseases that may pose particular risks in various areas. Many developing countries have high rates of tuberculosis, and HIV-infected persons are over 100 times more likely to get this infection than persons without HIV infection. Many areas pose a risk for malaria, and the standard precautions include avoidance of insect bites and certain preventive drugs that should not be a problem for HIV-infected persons. Visceral leishmaniasis (kala azar) is a disease transmitted by sandflies in many tropical countries that can be a major problem in patients with HIV infection. This includes South and Central America (New World) and Asia, Africa, and Southern Europe (Old World). The same applies to *Penicillium marneffei* in the Far East: Thailand, Hong Kong, China, Vietnam, Indonesia (Lancet 1994;344:110).

Despite these concerns, there is relatively little to support the claim that travel, even in late stages of HIV infection, is too dangerous due to exposures in other countries if simple precautions are taken.

Occupational Risks. The major occupational risks to persons with HIV infection are the health care field, child care providers, and occupations that require animal contact. In the health care field, the major risk is with tuberculosis exposure; this might also apply to employment in correctional facilities, shelters for the homeless, and volunteers for these sites. The specific risk depends to a large extent on the activities of the worker/volunteer and the prevalence of tuberculosis in the community. The major risk to providers of child care are *Cryptosporidia* and, to a lesser extent, *Cytomegalovirus*, hepatitis A, and giardiasis. The risk may be substantially reduced simply by good hygiene. Occupations requiring animal contact include veterinary work, and employment in farms, slaughter houses, or pet stores. The major risks are for *Cryptosporidia, Toxoplasma, Salmonella, Campylobacter,* and *Bartonella*. There is not good evidence that these occupations are sufficiently risky to avoid continued employment; the recommendation is to be aware of the risk and use appropriate precautions.

Most Common Presentations

Patients may present with known HIV serologic status; alternatively, they may present with complications of HIV infection without prior testing and without readily evident risk factors. Surveys show that up to one third of patients receive their first test within 2 months of an AIDS-defining illness (AIDS Clin Care 1997;9:1). Ten common findings at the time of initial evaluation follow.

1. Persistent Generalized Lymphadenopathy. This is defined as enlarged lymph nodes involving two noncontiguous sites other than inguinal nodes. Persistent generalized lymphadenopathy is a relatively common feature early in HIV infection reflecting the prominent role of the lymph system that harbors >95% of the total body burden of HIV. Studies of lymph nodes at this stage show high concentrations of HIV in germinal centers. Persistent generalized lymphadenopathy is important in the differential diagnosis of unexplained lymphadenopathy, and, in some cases, the lymph nodes are so firm or large that there is concern for alternative diagnoses such as lymphoma, secondary syphilis, or another diagnostic possibility. Mesenteric and periaortic nodes may be involved, but hilar and mediastinal nodes are not.

2. "Cytopenias." HIV infection is commonly complicated by anemia, leukopenia, and/or thrombocytopenia. Again, it is important to recognize HIV infection as a possible explanation for these findings in a patient who is being evaluated for other causes.

3. Pulmonary Symptoms Suggesting *Pneumocystis carinii* Pneumonia. The frequency of PCP as the initial AIDS-defining opportunistic infection has decreased from 74% in 1987 to 29% in 1996 reflecting the impact of PCP prophylaxis. Many cases now encountered are in patients who were unaware of their serologic status or noncompliant with PCP prophylaxis. The usual presentation is the combination of a nonproductive cough, dyspnea, and fever that often evolve over 2–4 weeks. Chest x-ray usually shows bilateral interstitial infiltrates with a highly characteristic ground-glass appearance; 10–30% of patients have normal x-rays. Additional diagnostic tests include blood gases to detect hypoxia and pulmonary function tests to detect abnormal diffusing capacity and/or LDH, which is elevated in 90% of cases. Diagnosis is usually established with induced sputum (sensitivity averages 60%) or bronchoalveolar lavage (BAL) from fiberoptic bronchoscopy (sensitivity >95%) (Am Rev Respir Dis 1992;145:1425).

4. Kaposi's Sarcoma. This diagnosis was previously second only to PCP in frequency as the initial AIDS-defining diagnosis based on CDC criteria of 1987 (MMWR 1987;36:35), but the frequency is rapidly decreasing, presumably reflecting changes in sexual practices of gay men. This condition is now ascribed to a newly detected herpes virus (Human Herpes Virus-8) that is transmitted by saliva or sex (N Engl J Med 1995; 332:1181; Nature Med 1996;2:918; N Engl J Med 1997;336:163). The typical lesion is a nodule or papule that is purple in light-skinned persons or dark brown or black in dark-skinned persons. It may be found on any part of the skin, mucous membranes, or visceral organs. Most patients will have multiple lesions on the skin, and the diagnosis can be established with a punch biopsy. A recent survey showed only 26% of primary care physicians diagnosed KS in a standardized patient with a typical lesion (JAMA 1995;274:1380).

5. Localized *Candida* Infections. Thrush is the most common presenting finding in patients with what was previously referred to as AIDS-related complex. In patients with HIV infection, this complication indicates advanced immunosuppression with a high probability of a serious opportunistic infection within 3 years in the absence of therapy. *Candida* esophagitis is a relatively late complication and is second only to PCP as the initial AIDS-defining opportunistic infection accounting for 11% of newly reported cases in 1995. The usual presentation is thrush with odynophagia. *Candida* vaginitis is common in women with or without HIV infection, although those with HIV infection are more likely to have infections that are recurrent or are refractory to therapy. (Nevertheless, CDC guidelines for managing recurrent or refractory cases of *Candida* vaginitis do not include HIV serology; MMWR 1993;42, RR-14:75).

6. Constitutional Symptoms. This refers to weight loss, night sweats, chronic fever, and/or chronic diarrhea found in advanced HIV infection. Fatigue is sometimes included, although this is a nonspecific symptom that may represent several other conditions. The chronicity of fever and diarrhea is defined by their presence for at least 30 days, which distinguishes these conditions from other common causes of diarrhea and fever that are unrelated to HIV. "Wasting syndrome" indicates HIV infection complicated by an otherwise unexplained loss of 10% of body weight. This accounted for 14% of newly reported AIDS cases in 1995 and is eventually encountered in 70–90%. The current impression is that rapid weight loss (>4 kg/4 mo) with anorexia is a sign of active infection; slower weight loss is often GI disease with diarrhea (N Engl J Med 1995;333:123; N Engl J Med 1995;333:83; Am J Clin Nutr 1993;58:417).

7. Bacterial Infections. Lower respiratory tract infection, presumably bacterial infections, are now the most common cause of death in patients with AIDS (N Engl J Med 1995;333: 845). In our experience at Johns Hopkins Hospital 46% of 385 patients with community-acquired pneumonia requiring hospitalization in 1993 had HIV infection; 35 (9%) of these patients were unaware of their HIV status (Am J Respir Crit Care Med 1995;152:1309). The rates of pneumococcal pneumonia and pneumococcal bacteremia are 150- to 300-fold higher in persons with HIV infection compared to expected rates [JAMA 191;265: 3275; JID 1990;162:1012; CID 1995;21(suppl 1):S277]. Other bacterial pathogens and conditions they cause that appear with substantially increased rates are pneumonia from *H. influenzae* (including type B), *Legionella,* and *P. aeruginosa; S. aureus* causing line sepsis, endocarditis (IV drug use), pyomyositis, etc.; salmonellosis; *Clostridium difficile*-associated diarrhea/colitis reflecting increased use of antibacterial agents; line sepsis (rates with

Hickman catheters as high as 60%/year) and sinusitis (microbial cause usually unknown and often refractory to standard treatment). Less common bacterial pathogens are *Nocardia asteroides, Rhodococcus equi,* and *Bartonella henselae/quintana*. The points to emphasize are *(a)* bacterial infections are relatively common in patients with HIV infection despite their infrequency in the tabulation of AIDS-defining diagnoses and *(b)* bacterial infections may occur relatively early in HIV infection, reflecting increased virulence of these pathogens compared with the more classic opportunistic pathogens and the concurrent risk of HIV infection and bacterial infections associated with injection drug use.

8. Tuberculosis. The seroprevalence rate of HIV in patients with active tuberculosis in the U.S. is 4–40% depending on geographic area. The frequency of TB among patients with AIDS averages 5% with highest rates in New York state—10.6%, Illinois—7%, Florida—5.9%, Georgia—5.6%, and Texas—4.7% (J AIDS 1996;12:293). The current CDC recommendations are that all patients with active tuberculosis should have HIV serology, and all patients with HIV infection should have a PPD.

9. STDs. The seroprevalence of HIV infection in 552,665 patients from 80 STD clinics obtained from 1988 to 1992 showed: gay men—33%, heterosexual men—3%, women—2%, heterosexual injection drug users—10% (J AIDS 1995;9:514). Genital ulcer disease (syphilis, herpes simplex, and chancroid) appears to be especially important in HIV transmission (Lancet 1989;2: 403). Nonulcerative diseases such as gonococcal infection, chlamydia infection, and bacterial vaginosis also appear to promote HIV transmission (JID 1991;163:233; AIDS 1993;7:95; STD 1992; 19:61). All patients with STDs should have HIV serology with informed consent according to current CDC guidelines.

10. Neurologic Syndromes. HIV causes numerous neurologic syndromes, but the most common are HIV-associated dementia in 20–30% and peripheral neuropathy in 20–30%. The former is characterized in early stages by difficulty concentrating, mental slowing, and memory loss. Differentiation from depression may be difficult. Findings that indicate probable HIV-associated dementia include the following: history of progressive cognitive deterioration (with clear consciousness), cognitive deterioration in neurologic assessment with either normal or diffuse CNS signs, significant deterioration with neuropsychological assessment, and exclusion of alternative causes: stable psychiatric medication regimen, no metabolic disorder (uremia, sepsis, liver failure, intoxication), and exclusion of opportunistic infections and neurosyphilis (Neurology 1994;44: 1892). Sensory neuropathy generally presents with pain and paresthesias affecting the feet (Medicine 1987;66:407).

Physical Examination

The physical examination in patients with HIV infection should include attention to those anatomic sites that are likely to show significant changes and prove useful in management, including staging. Especially important are lymph node evaluation, funduscopic examination, oral cavity evaluation, careful skin examination, abdominal examination for hepatosplenomegaly, genital examination for STDs, pelvic examination in women, and neuropsychological testing (Table 10). The following components of the standard evaluation are often neglected.

Gynecologic Complications. Women with HIV infection have high rates of gynecologic complications, including recurrent or refractory vaginal candidiasis as a common early manifestation. Prevalence rates of cervical dysplasia are increased 8- to 11-fold. An association between cervical neoplasia and declining immune function has been noted, and rapidly progressive cervical cancer in young women with HIV infection has been reported (JAMA 1991;266:2253; Obstet Gynecol 1991;78:84). Pelvic inflammatory disease in HIV infected women is associated with higher fever, longer time to defervesence and longer lengths of hospitilization (Ob Gyn 1997;89:65; Lancet 1997; 349: 1265). The CDC recommends a gynecologic evaluation and Pap smear with the initial evaluation, a repeat Pap smear 6 months later, and then annual tests if results are normal (MMWR 1990; 39:47). Women with HIV infection also need specialized counseling as appropriate for HIV testing and on care of children, reproduction, and abortion.

Neurologic Examination. The neurologic examination should include evaluation for HIV-associated dementia (formerly referred to as AIDS dementia complex), which is noted in 20–30% of patients but almost exclusively appears in the late stages with advanced immunosuppression. Relevant observa-

Table 10. Major Diagnostic Considerations by Organ System[a]

Conditions	CD4 > 300/mm³	CD4 < 200/mm³
Lymphadenopathy	PGL (syphilis, lymphoma, KS, TB)	PGL (CMV, TB, KS, MA)
Eye (fundi)		
Exudate + hemorrhage		CMV retinitis
Cotton wool spots	HIV retinopathy	HIV retinopathy
Oral		
White patches	Thrush, OHL	Thrush, OHL
Ulcers	HSV, aphthous ulcers	HSV, aphthous ulcers, (CMV)
Red-purple nodular lesions	KS	KS
Esophagus (dysphagia)		*Candida* CMV, aphthous ulcers (HSV)
Abdomen		
Diarrhea	*Salmonella, C. difficile, Campylobacter, Shigella,* viral agents, cryptosporidiosis	Cryptosporidia, microsporidia, MA, CMV, adverse drug reaction, *C. difficile,* AIDS enteropathy (small bowel overgrowth, histoplasmosis, isospora, cyclospora, lymphoma)
Hepatomegaly and/or abnormal LFTs	Hepatitis (usually HBV or HCV) Adverse drug reaction	Hepatitis, (HBV or HCV), CMV, MA, lymphoma, HIV, fatty liver 2* malnutrition; cholangiopathy-cryptosporidia, CMV, idiopathic, (microsporidia)
Splenomegaly	HIV	Lymphoma, MA, histoplasmosis, HIV, cirrhosis

Skin		
Purple-black nodular lesions	KS (bacillary angiomatosis, prurigo nodularis)	KS (bacillary angiomatosis, prurigo nodularis)
Vesicles	Herpes simplex, herpes zoster	Herpes simplex, herpes zoster (CMV)
Maculopapular lesions	Adverse drug reaction, syphilis	Adverse drug reaction, syphilis
Plaques, scaling lesions	Seborrhea (psoriasis, eczema)	Seborrhea (psoriasis, eczema)
Umbilicated papules	Molluscum	Molluscum (cryptococcus)
Petechiae, purpura	ITP	ITP
Nodules		Cryptococcus, histoplasmosis, pruritis nodularis
Lungs		
Pneumonia	*S. pneumoniae*, (*H. influenzae*, TB, aspiration, atypical agents)	PCP, bacterial infections (TB, MA, KS, CMV, cryptococcus, histoplasmosis, lymphocytic interstitial pneumonia)
Cavity, nodules	TB (*S. aureus* with IV drug users)	TB (cryptococcus, nocardia, KS, lymphoma, MA, *M. kansasii*, atypical PCP, *Rhodococcus*, *Aspergillus*)
Neurological		
Aseptic meningitis	Neurosyphilis, viral	Cryptococcus
Chronic meningitis	Tuberculosis, neurosyphilis	Cryptococcus, tuberculosis, neurosyphilis
Dementia	Trauma, tumor, depression, hypothyroid	HIV-associated dementia
Constitutional symptoms (FUO, weight loss, etc.)	Lymphoma, TB	MA, CMV, histoplasmosis, HIV, cryptococcosis, PCP, lymphoma

[a] *CMV*, cytomegalovirus; *PCP*, *P. carinii* pneumonia; *MA*, *M. avium*; *TB*, tuberculosis; *OHL*, oral hairy leukoplakia; *PGL*, peripheral generalized lymphadenopathy; *HSV*, herpes simplex virus; *ADC*, AIDS dementia complex.

[b] Conditions in parentheses indicate less likely diagnosis.

tions are (a) the earliest symptoms of cognitive defects are problems with concentration and memory; (b) the earliest subjective motor dysfunction is imbalance, incoordination, or difficulty with complex motor tasks; (c) the most frequent findings with neuropsychological testing are slowed verbal responses and difficulties with complex sequencing, problem solving, performance with time pressure, and visual-motor integration such as "pathfinding;" (d) neurologic testing often shows problems with rapid alternating movements, hyperreflexia, and ataxia; and (e) neuroradiologic scan studies usually show cerebral atrophy with or without abnormal white matter. The standard Mini-Mental test is insensitive; timed tests such as the HIV Dementia Scale are preferred (Neurology 1991;41:1905; Arch Neurol 1994; 51:689; Arch Gen Psychiatry 1991;48:141).

Psychiatric Evaluation. Our experience indicates over 50% of newly diagnosed HIV-infected patients have a major mental illness other than substance abuse or personality disorder. About 20–30% develop a major depression at some time during the disease, and this bears little relationship to any prior history of depression or to a family history of depression. Depression is most common at advanced stages of HIV infection. Most patients respond well to tricyclic antidepressants. Delirium is also common and is distinguished from dementia by acute onset, "waxing and waning" mental state, disrupted sleep, speech that is often incoherent, and reduced awareness. Most patients with delirium respond well to low-dose neuroleptic agents.

Nutritional Assessment. Nutritional assessment is important because wasting is such a common feature of late-stage disease. Contributing factors are increased metabolic requirements, reduced intake (depression, dementia, anorexia, taste perversion, oral/esophageal lesions, nausea, drug reaction), and malabsorption (with or without diarrhea). Patients with weight loss need a medical evaluation. Rapid weight loss with >4 kg over 4 months usually indicates an intercurrent infection (Am J Clin Nutr 1992;55:455). A more gradual weight loss may be due to anorexia and/or GI disease. Metabolic studies of HIV-infected patients with wasting show total energy expenditure is not high so that weight loss must be ascribed to reduced food intake. The prevention of weight loss or promotion of weight gain must be done with increased energy supply. Various tactics include consultation with a nutritionist, appetite stimulants (Megace or Marinol), nutritional supplements, or a variety of newer therapies that are gaining popular appeal: thalidomide, testosterone ± megace, anabolic steroids, and serostin (growth hormone). A distinction should be made between weight gain that is fat and weight gain from increases in lean body mass. A potential advantage of testosterone, anabolic steroids, and growth hormone is the increase achieved in lean body mass. The role of routine nutritional consultation in patients with stable weight is not established. Prolonged (>3 wk) parenteral hyperalimentation has no established value in proper studies and should probably be reserved for patients with devastating protein-calorie malnutrition caused by uncontrollable diarrhea associated with cryptosporidiosis.

Ophthalmologic Examination. CMV retinitis complicates the course of about 20% of patients with HIV infection. Initial lesions are often in the periphery and cannot be visualized by routine funduscopic examination. CMV retinitis usually progresses to blindness in the absence of treatment, and therapy usually halts progression at least temporarily. AIDS patients with CMV retinitis have a mean CD4 cell count of $20/mm^3$, and only 1% have a count above $100/mm^3$. Routine exam by an ophthalmologist detects CMV retinitis in about 15% of AIDS patients with CD4 counts $\leq 50/mm^3$. Based on these observations some recommend a routine ophthalmologic consultation at 6-month intervals for patients with a CD4 count below $100/mm^3$ and at 3- to 4-month intervals with CD4 counts $<50/mm^3$. This is also advised for patients with CMV disease at other anatomical sites. The importance of such screening for early detection of CMV retinitis is not established because the need for early intervention is not established.

Laboratory Testing

The usual laboratory tests performed with initial evaluation are designed to (a) ensure confirmation of HIV infection; (b) stage the disease; (c) identify latent pathogens that will influence subsequent strategies for treatment and prophylaxis; and (d) determine general health status. Specific guidelines are summarized in Table 11.

Table 11. Routine Laboratory Tests in Patients with HIV Infection

Test	Cost	Frequency	Comment
HIV serology	Ave $40	IX	• Repeat test for patients who have: 1) No identified risks, 2) No confirmation, 3) Prior test with nonstandard method • Plasma HIV RNA is confirmatory if positive
CBC	$6–8	Every 3–4 months	• Repeat more frequently with marrow suppression
CD4 count	$40–150	Every 3–4 months	• Standard method to monitor immunocompetency • Routine testing is unnecessary for untreated patients with CD4 count $<50/mm^3$ • Outlier results should be confirmed due to large variations in test results
Plasma HIV RNA	$43–290	Every 3–4 months and 2–4 weeks after new therapy	• Standard method to evaluate prognosis and response to therapy • Recommendation is baseline tests ×2 separated by ≥2 weeks; with initiation of treatment or change in treatment the test should be repeated at 4 weeks to determine initial response (alpha slope) and at 8 wks to determine maximal effect (beta slope) • Testing should be done using same lab, same technique, an assay with a lower threshold of ≤500 copies/ml, at a time of clinical stability, and ≥1 mo from immunizations
Serum chemistries	$10–15	Annual or more frequent	• Major interest is hepatic function test due to high rates of chronic hepatitis • Monitoring more frequently is necessary with use of nephrotoxic or hepatotoxic drugs including most antiretroviral agents
Anti HBc	$10–15	XI in candidates for HBV vaccime	• Candidate for HBV vaccine: Seronegative persons at high risk—injection drug users, sexually active gay men, prostitutes, STD patients, >1 sexual partner past 6 mo, household or sex contract with HBsAg carrier

Anti HCV and HBsAg	$40–60	XI in patient with unexplained abnormal LFTs	
Toxoplasma IgG	$12–15	XI (see comments)	• Screen all patients and repeat in seronegatives if: 1) CD4 count <100/mm^3 and patient does not take TMP-SMX prophylaxis and 2) symptoms suggesting toxoplasmosis
PPD	$1	XI (see comment)	• Indicated if no history of positive PPD or treatment of TB • Repeat annually if high risk of TB and with exposure
Chest x-ray	$40–100	See comment	• Commonly advocated at baseline but prior study of 1065 HIV-infected patients showed virtually no useful information (Arch Intern Med 1996;156:191) • Indicated in patients with positive PPD, history of chest disease, or pulmonary symptoms
PAP smear	$25–40	Baseline, 6 months, then annually	• Repeat results reported as inadequate • Refer to gynecologist for atypia or greater on the Bethesda score
CMV serology	$10–15	See comment	• Advocated for detection of latent CMV primarily in low-risk patients to: 1) permit counseling for CMV prevention (same as HIV), 2) to assist in differential diagnosis of possible CMV disease, and 3) to guide use of CMV-antibody negative blood or leukocyte-reduced blood products
VDRL or RPR	$5–16	Annual in sexually-active pts	• Positives must have FTA confirmation: up to 6% of HIV-infected patients have false-positive screening tests (CID 1994;*19*:1040; Am J Med 1995;99:55) • True positives require CSF analysis (Am Intern Med 1990;113:872)

HIV Serology. Guidelines for HIV serology in terms of indications, interpretation, and use of alternative tests are summarized on pages 1–9. It is emphasized here that documentation of a positive HIV serology is indicated except for patients who refuse the test. CD4 counts may serve as a surrogate marker for advanced HIV infection in patients with possible HIV-related complications when serology results are delayed or serology is refused. The CBC can be used to detect lymphopenia (<1000/mm^3), which is supportive. A CD4 count is obviously more specific since relatively few conditions in medicine other than HIV cause severe depletion of CD4 cells; acute corticosteroid therapy may cause this. HIV serology is clearly more sensitive and specific, although there are relatively few medical conditions associated with counts <300/mm^3.

Complete Blood Count (CBC). This is a standard component of the initial evaluation in virtually any health assessment and is especially important in patients with HIV infection because anemia, leukopenia, and thrombocytopenia are common complications. A separate platelet count is usually not required with the standard Coulter counter analysis used by most labs because this is a routine determination.

CD4 Cell Count. This is a pivotal test for evaluation of any patient with HIV infection to stage the disease and provide guidelines for differential diagnosis of patient complaints; it dictates therapeutic decisions regarding antiviral treatment and prophylaxis for opportunistic pathogens. Mean levels in healthy controls for most laboratories are 800–1050/mm^3 with a range representing two standard deviations of about 450–1400/mm^3 (Ann Intern Med 1993;119:55). There is substantial variation in the test results owing to technology, diurnal variations, and possible influence of intercurrent illnesses. These variations are more likely to be profound in early-stage disease with high counts rather than late-stage disease. Diurnal changes show lowest levels at 12:30 p.m. and peak values at 8:30 p.m. The average diurnal change in HIV-infected persons with counts of 200–500 is 60/mm^3 (J AIDS 1990;3:144). Marked laboratory variations reflect the fact that the count represents the product of three variables: white blood cell count, percent lymphocytes, and percent lymphocytes that bear the CD4 receptor. High-quality laboratories participating in ACTG trials showed the average within-subject coefficient of variation was 25% (J Infect Dis 1994; 169:28). A comparison of four labs performing tests on 24 patients showed the average difference between high and low values was 108/mm^3; 14 of the 24 had results that would lead to different therapeutic decisions (CID 1995;21:1121). Standards for quality assurance have recently been published by the CDC (MMWR 1997;46 RR-2). Methods to reduce variations are to use the same laboratory and maintain consistency in the time of blood draws. Some clinicians prefer to utilize the CD4 percent because this reduces variation to one measurement (J AIDS 1989; 2:114). Corresponding CD4 cell counts are the following:

CD4 Cell Count	%CD4
>500	>29
200–500/mm^3	14–28
<200/mm^3	<14

Medical conditions that cause modest decreases in CD4 cell count include acute CMV infection, hepatitis B infection, tuberculosis, some bacterial infections, and major surgery. Corticosteroid administration may have a profound effect with decreases from 900 to <300/mm^3 after acute administration of high doses; chronic administration has a much less pronounced effect. Strenuous exercise may lower absolute lymphocyte subsets (MMWR 1997;46:1). Coinfection with HTLV-1 and splenectomy may be responsible for a deceptively high CD4 count. Factors that have minimal effect are gender, age in adults, risk category, psychological stress, physical stress, and pregnancy (Ann Intern Med 1993;119:55).

CD4 counts of 500/mm^3 are within normal range for most laboratories, but this represents a substantial reduction in immune competence. With 350/mm^3 there is severe damage that may be irreversible. Most complications of HIV infection occur with CD4 counts <200/mm^3 and many are associated with mean CD4 counts of <50/mm^3. The CD4 count consequently represents an important test for evaluating immunocompetence and determining probabilities of various complications.

In some areas of the world it may not be possible to obtain a CD4 count, and in some clinical settings in the U.S. these results may be delayed. WHO has proposed use of the total lymphocyte count when CD4 counts are unavailable. A lymphocyte count below 1000/mm^3 is strongly predictive of a CD4 count below 200/mm^3 (JAMA 1993;269:622).

Quantitative HIV RNA. This assay has revolutionized patient evaluation and therapeutic monitoring. Most important were studies of the Multicenter AIDS Cohort Study (MACS), which is a prospective longitudinal study of HIV infection in gay men that was initiated in 1984. When technology was developed to quantitate plasma HIV RNA, stored frozen sera from this cohort were analyzed for correlation with clinical outcome according to assessments at 6-month intervals for the ensuing decade. This and other studies now provide the database for current concepts regarding quantitative HIV RNA with the following conclusions (Ann Intern Med 1995;122:573; Science 1996; 272:1167; JID 1996;174:696; JID 1996;174:704):

- Natural history: The acute retroviral syndrome is associated with high-level HIV RNA ($\geq 10^5$ copies/mL); this decreases abruptly with immune response, and a "set point" is established at about 6 months. This set point is relatively stable for years in the absence of antiretroviral therapy. The concentration correlates directly with the rate of clinical progression based on CD4 slope, time to an AIDS-defining complication, and survival (Table 12).
- The viral burden analysis was done with heparinized blood specimens; the numbers provided should be doubled to approximate the adjustment for the deleterious effect of heparin on RNA copy number.
- Therapeutic monitoring: Antiretroviral therapy in patients with HIV shows two decay curves: The alpha slope is the

Table 12. Viral Burden Analysis

Viral Burden (copies/mL)*	No. Pts.	Relative Hazard: AIDS	Relative Hazard: Death	Survival (median)	CD4 Slope
<500	112	1.0	1.0	>10 yrs	−36
500–3,000	229	2.4	2.8	>10 yrs	−45
3,000–10,000	347	4.4	5.0	>10 yrs	−55
10,000–30,000	357	7.6	9.9	7.5 yrs	−65
>30,000	386	13	18.5	4.4 yrs	−76

MACS Data (Mellors J et al. Ann Intern Med, in press)

initial decline noted within 2–4 wks of treatment. This primarily reflects decreases in free plasma HIV RNA and HIV in acutely infected CD4 cells. The beta slope is a modest incremental decrease beyond the alpha slope over 4–6 months. This primarily reflects the antiviral effect on latently infected CD4 cells, macrophages, and released HIV from follicular dendridic cells. The implications of these observations are that the impact of new or changed therapy can be determined within 2–4 weeks and the total impact of treatment can be determined at 4–6 months.

- Goal of therapy: The goal of antiretroviral therapy that has evolved from recent therapeutic trials is "no detectable virus" using an assay that has a detection threshold of ≤500 copies/mL. The rationale for this objective is that (1) viral burden reflects HIV replication (2) HIV replication accounts for disease progression, and (3) limited replication reduces mutations that are responsible for evolution of drug resistance. There are rapidly evolving data to support these conclusions. Data from therapeutic trials using quantitative HIV monitoring show (1) reductions in viral burden are associated with CD4 count increases (a 1-log decrease usually equates to an increase in CD4 count of 50–85/mm^3); (2) reduced viral burden correlates with a reduction in clinical progression, in terms of AIDS-defining complications, and survival (i.e., treatment appears to reestablish the set point); (3) there appears to be a limited response in terms of reconstitution of immune function with maximal mean CD4 increases of 100–150/mm^3; and (4) these are marked differences between regimens; in general, monotherapy with nucleoside analogues results in mean decreases of 0.5–0.8 log that are not sustained >6–12 mo, double nucleoside treatment produces mean decreases of 0.8–1.5 log that are usually not sustained >12 mo, and protease inhibitors plus two nucleosides produce mean decreases of >2 logs with no detectable virus in >50% for periods of ≥ 1 year.
- Cost: $47–292 (based on surveys of multiple AIDS care providers; the $47 assay was a "bundled rate")
- Recommendations: Adapted from International AIDS Society USA (Nature Med 1996;2:625)

Frequency: Baseline ×2 separated by 2 wks; monitor every 3–4 months; for therapeutic monitoring after new or changed treatment: 2–4 wks (alpha slope) and 4–6 mo (beta slope)

CD4 count: Quantitative HIV RNA does not supplant the need for CD4 monitoring at 3- to 4-mo intervals since they measure different effects of HIV infections. The CD4 count measures the extent of immune suppression, dictates the need for OI prophylaxis, dictates the differential diagnosis of clinical presentations, and represents an independent indicator of prognosis.

Quality assurance: Quantitative HIV RNA should be done by the same lab using the same technique at periods of clinical stability and at a time ≥ after acute infection or immunization.

Interpretation: Changes >50% (0.3 log) generally are considered significant.

Factors that increase viral burden: (1) Progressive disease; (2) infection (active TB, pneumococcal pneumonia, HSV, etc) (3) immunization (for 2–4 wks) and (4) failed antiretroviral therapy.

Syphilis Serology. Screening tests (VDRL or RPR) should be performed with the initial evaluation and repeated annually in patients who are sexually active. False-negative and false-positive tests have been reported in patients with HIV infection (J Infect Dis 1990;162:862; J Infect Dis 1992;165:1020; AIDS 1991; 5:419), but these are rare (Ann Intern Med 1990;113:872). Patients with a positive screening test should have a confirmatory fluorescent treponemal antibody absorption test. All patients with HIV infection and positive syphilis serology should undergo a lumbar puncture.

Serum Chemistry Panel. This test is considered to be of limited value in a general health screen (Ann Intern Med 1987; 106:403) but is advocated for the initial evaluation of patients with HIV infection caused by high rates of concurrent illnesses, including hepatitis; this also serves as a baseline value for patients who may have multisystem complications and require polypharmacy.

Table 13. Quantitative HIV RNA

	Roche	Chiron	Organon
Contact	Patient Assistance 999-837-8727	Technical Inquiry Customer Service Testing Laboratory 800-434-2447	919-620-2000 Mike Cronin Stuart Geiger
Technique	RT-PCR	bDNA	NASBA
Range of assay (Copies/ml)	Roche Amplicor HIV-1 400 to 750,000 copies/ml	bDNA Version 2.0 500–1,000 to 10^6 copies/ml	NASBA Version 1 400–10,000,000 copies/ml
Threshold ``Next generation test''	20 copies/ml	20 copies/ml	20–40 copies/ml
Specimens			
Volume	0.5 ml	0.5 ml	1.0–2.0 ml
Tubes	EDTA (lavender top)	EDTA (lavender top)	EDTA, heparin, whole blood, any body fluid
Requirement	Separate plasma <6 hr and freeze prior to shipping	Separate plasma <4 hr and freeze prior to shipping	Separate plasma <48 hrs and place in lysis buffer >48 hrs—freeze prior to shipping
Shipping	Frozen plasma aon dry ice for overnight courier	Frozen plasma on dry ince for overnight courier	Lysis buffer supplied by Organon Teknika

Hepatitis Serology. The choice of diagnostic test depends on the clinical situation. Patients considered candidates for hepatitis B vaccination (injection drug use, sexually active gay men, heterosexual men and women with sexually transmitted diseases or more than one sex partner in the past 6 months, and household or sex contacts of a HBsAg carrier) should have serologic testing to determine established immunity using anti-HBc (N Engl J Med 1997;336:196). Serologic screening is considered cost effective since the vaccination price is about $160 for the standard three-dose regimen, the rate of positive tests for Hepatitis B markers indicating immunity in gay men or injection drug users is 60–80%, and the cost of serologic testing is usually $12–20. Patients with abnormal liver function tests with the serum chemistry panel need evaluation for active hepatitis infection with either HBV or HCV. The appropriate tests are HBV surface antigen (HBsAg) and antibodies to HCV (anti-HCV).

Toxoplasmosis Serology. IgG for *T. gondii* is advocated: (1) at the initial screen to determine latent infection, (2) in previously seronegative or untested patients who become candidates for toxoplasmosis prophylaxis using agents other than TMP-SMX (given for PCP prophylaxis) due to a CD4 count $<100/mm^3$, and (3) in previously seronegative or untested patients who have possible CNS toxoplasmosis. Seronegative patients should be warned to avoid unnecessary contact such as rare meat and litter pans of kittens. Seroprevalence for adults in the US is usually 10–30%; sensitivity of the test in patients with CNS toxoplasmosis is 85–100%.

Cytomegalovirus Serology. This is an arbitrary inclusion sometimes advocated with initial evaluation to detect latent CMV infection in patients with a low risk of harboring CMV. Seroprevalence of CMV in healthy adults in the US is 50–70%; it is >90% in gay men, IDUs, and hemophiliacs. Possible applications are the use of this information in differential diagnosis of possible CMV disease, to identify candidates for CMV prophylaxis (although this is not a current recommendation), and to identify persons who should have leukocyte filtration with transfusions.

PPD Skin Test. The CDC recommends routine testing with PPD (using the standard Mantoux test) 5TU units with interpretation at 48–72 hours by a health care professional. A recent prospective study of 1130 HIV-infected persons followed a median of 53 months showed the rate of active TB was 0.5/100 in those who remained PPD negative compared with 3.2/100 in those with baseline positive PPD tests and 4.7/100 in those who seroconverted (Ann Intern Med 1997;126:123). There is consensus that the PPD test should have a high priority, but the utility and reliability of anergy testing are debated. Many authorities no longer recommend it due to lack of standardization of reagents and inconsistent results with repeat tests in HIV-infected patients (Arch Intern Med 1993;155:2111). If done, anergy testing should include two skin test reagents: *Candida albicans,* tetanus toxoid, and/or mumps (MMWR 1991;49 RR-5:1). The definition of a positive PPD in HIV-infected patients is ≥ 5 mm induration; with the anergy screen it is any induration.

Pap Smear. The CDC recommends a gynecologic evaluation with pelvic examination and Pap smear in women with HIV infection at initial evaluation, a repeat Pap smear 6 months later, and then annually if results are normal (MMWR 1990;39: 47). Current recommendations for managing results are shown in Table 14.

Chest X-Ray. A chest x-ray is recommended for detection of asymptomatic tuberculosis and also as a baseline test for patients who have high rates of pulmonary disease. This baseline

Table 14. Management and Abnormal Pap Test Results: Recommendations of the Agency for Health Care Policy and Research and the National Cancer Institute

Results	Action
Inadequate	Repeat
Atypia	Repeat pap smear every 4–6 mo × 2 years to achieve 3 consecutive negative smears *or* colposcopy
Inflammation	Evaluation for infection, treat and repeat pap smear in 2–3 mo
Low-grade squamous intraepithelial lesion	Colcoposcopy and biopsy or follow-up paps smear every 4–6 months with colposcopy plus biopsy if abnormalities persist
High-grade squamous Intraepithelial lesions or squamous cell carcinoma	Colposcopy and biopsy

JAMA 1994;271:1866.

screening test is endorsed by the USPHS/IDSA Guidelines. A review of screening chest x-rays in 1065 HIV-infected persons at 0-, 3-, 6-, and 12-month intervals showed only 2% were abnormal, and this technique detected only 11 of 55 patients who developed pulmonary complications within 2 months of the x-ray. The yield was low in groups at high risk for TB and those with low CD4 counts. The authors conclude that chest x-rays as a screening test in asymptomatic HIV-infected persons with a negative PPD are unwarranted (Arch Intern Med 1996;156: 191).

Glucose-6-Phosphate Dehydrogenase Level. Glucose-6-phosphate dehydrogenase (G-6-PD) deficiency is a genetic disease that predisposes to hemolytic anemia after exposure to oxidant drugs. There are more than 300 variants that are inherited on the X chromosome. The most common form is GdA, which is found in 10% of black men and 1–2% of black women; the most serious form is GdMED found predominantly in men from the Mediterranean area (Italians, Greeks, Sephardic Jews, Arabs) and men from India and Southeast Asia. In most cases, the hemolysis is mild and self-limited because only the older red cells are involved and the bone marrow can compensate. The most important exception is GdMED, which may cause life-threatening hemolysis. The severity of anemia also depends on concentration of the drug in the red cells and the oxidant potential; the most likely offending agents used in patients with HIV infection are dapsone and primaquine and less likely are sulfonamides. During hemolysis, G-6-PD levels are usually normal because the susceptible red cells have been destroyed so that testing must be delayed for about 1 month after a drug holiday. Methemoglobin levels will be elevated. Options for testing are to (1) obtain this test at baseline; (2) screen patients at high risk (African-American men and men of Mediterranean descent); (3) delay testing until oxidant drugs are indicated; or (4) delay until hemolysis is suspected (with measurement of methemoglobin acutely and level of G-6-PD after a drug holiday). It should be emphasized that most patients with low levels tolerate oxidant drugs well; it would be a mistake to consider, for example, trimethoprim-sulfamethoxazole (TMP-SMX) or dapsone to be absolutely contraindicated in an African-American male with an abnormally low G-6-PD level.

4—Prevention: Opportunistic Infections

(see Table 15) USPH/IDSA Guidelines (MMWR 1995;44 RR-8; CID 1995;21, Supplement 1, Ann Intern Med 1996; 124:348 and 1997 USPH/IDSA Guidelines—Draft 5/97)

The US Public Health Service and the Infectious Disease Society of America provided guidelines on strategies to reduce the frequency of opportunistic infections that were published in 1995. The Task Force consisted of 65 experts in the field under leadership of Henry Masur (NIH), Jonathan Kaplan (CDC), and King Holmes (Univ. Washington). This group reconvened in November 1996 to provide revisions; the recommendations below are based on the 1995 document and the draft version of the 1997 document. These recommendations are presented as follows:

Table 15: Recommendations for Prevention of Opportunistic Infection

Table 16: Strength and Quality of Opportunistic Infection

Table 17: Recommendations for OI Prophylaxis During Pregnancy

Table 18: Recommendations for Vaccines

Table 15. Prevention of Opportunistic Infections: Antimicrobial Prophylaxis: Recommendation of USPH/IDSA (MMWR 44 RR-8, 1995 and draft revisions 1/13/97)

Disease	Indications	Preferred Regimen (cost/mo)	Comment
STRONGLY RECOMMENDED AS STANDARD OF CARE			
Tuberculosis	PPD + (≥5 mm induration) Prior positive PPD without INH prophylaxis High risk exposure	INH 300 mg/d + pyridoxine 50 mg/d or 900 mg 2×/wk + 50 mg/d ($0.60/mo)	• Efficacy established • Alternative (INH resistance or toxicity): rifampin 600 mg/d × 12 mo • Some advocate life-long prophylaxis
P. carinii pneumonia	Prior PCP CD4 < 200 Thrush or FUO	TMP-SMX 1 DS/d ($2.10/mo)	• Efficacy established: cost effective, reduced morbidity and mortality • Alternatives: TMP-SMX 1 SS (single strength) daily or 1 DS 3 days/wk; dapsone 100 mg/d; regimens for toxoplasmosis (see below) or aerosolized pentamidine 300 mg/mo
Toxoplasmosis	CD4 < 100 *plus* positive serology (IgG)	TMP-SMX 1 DS/d ($2.10/mo)	• Efficiacy established • Main issue is use of alternative regimens in patients with TMP-SMX intolerance: dapsone 50 mg/d + pyrimethamine 50 mg/wk + leucovorin 25 mg/wk *or* dapsone 200 mg/wk + pyrimethamine 75 mg/wk + leucovorin 25 mg/wk
M. avium	CD4 < 50	Clarithromycin 500 mg bid ($181/mo) Azithromycin 1200 mg 1×/wk ($94/mo)	• Efficacy established • Clarithromycin and azithromycin are superior to rifabutin for MAC prophylaxis • Alternatives are rifabutin 300 mg/d or rifabutin 300 mg/d + azithromycin 1200 mg q week

			• A disadvantage of macrolides is possible resistace to clarithromycin which is the favored agent for treatment or established infection
Streptococcus pneumoniae	All patients	Pneumococcal vaccine 0.5 mL IM ×1	• Response is reduced in patients with CD4 counts <200/mm^3
Varicella	Exposure to chicken pox or zoster	Varicella-zoster immune globulin (VZIG), 625 units (5 Vials) IM <96 h post exposure	• Acyclovir 800 mg 5×/d × 21 days is an alternative, but efficacy is not established
NOT RECOMMENDED FOR MOST PATIENTS			
CMV	CD4 < 50	Oral ganciclovir 1000 mg tid ($1404/mo)	• Efficacy shown in the Syntex study, but not in CPCRA 023 • Concerns are cost, promotion of ganciclovir resistance and preliminary state of data. Many authorities feel that indications for CMV prophylaxis will be redefined by use of PCR to detect CMV in blood or quantitative PCR
Candida	CD4 < 100	Fluconazole 100–200 mg/d ($206–337/mo)	• Efficacy established for prevention of cryptococcosis and *Candida* esophagitis (and thrush) • Concerns are cost, lack of evidence for prolongation of survival and promotion of infection with azole-resistant *Candida* spp.

Table 15. *(continued)*

Disease	Indications	Preferred Regimen (cost/mo)	Comment
Cryptococcosis	CD4 < 50	Fluconazole 100–200 mg/d	• Efficacy established • Alternative is itraconazole 200 mg/d • Concerns are failure to show survival advantage, promotion of azole resistant *Candida* and C. neoformans drug interactions, infrequency of cryptococcosis, and cost • Doses of 400 mg/week are effective
Histoplasmosis	CD4 < 100 plus endemic area	Itraconazole capsules 200 mg/d	• Efficacy established • Itraconazole capsules at this dose does not effectively suppress Candida infections
Coccidioidomycosis	CD4 < 50 plus endemic area	Fluconazole 200 mg/d	• Efficacy and prophylaxis is unknown
Bacteria	Neutropenia ANC < 500/ml	G-CSF 5–10 μg/kg SC qd × 2–4 wks or GM-CSF	
RECOMMENDED FOR CONSIDERATION			
Hepatitis B	Susceptible—anti-HBc neg	Recombivax HB 10 μg IM × 3 *or* Engerix-B 20 μg IM × 3	
Influenza	All patients	Influenza vaccine	

Table 16. Strength and Quality of Opportunistic Infection Prophylaxis

US Public Health Service—Infectious Disease Society of America Guidelines for Prevention of Opportunistic Infections (MMWR44 RR-8, 1995)
Guidelines are categorized on the strength (Category A–E) and quality (Category I–III) of the supporting evidence
Categories reflecting the strength of each recommendation for or against the use of a product or measure for the prevention of opportunistic infection in HIV-infected persons

Category	Definition
A	Both strong evidence and substantial clinical benefit support a recommendation for use.
B	Moderate evidence—or strong evidence for only limited benefit—supports a recommendation for use.
C	Poor evidence supports a recommendation for or against use.
D	Moderate evidence supports a recommendation against use.
E	Good evidence supports a recommendation against use.

Categories reflecting the quality of evidence forming the basis for recommendations regarding the use of a product or measure for the prevention of opportunistic infection in HIV-infected persons

Category	Definition
I	Evidence from at least one properly randomized, controlled trial
II	Evidence from at least one well-designed clinical trial without randomization, from cohort or case-controlled analytic studies (preferably from more than one center), or from multiple time-series studies or dramatic results from uncontrolled experiments
III	Evidence from opinions of respected authorities based on clinical experience, descriptive studies, or reports of expert committees

NOTE: Modified from Gross et al. Clin Infect Dis 1994;18:421.

Table 16. *(continued)*

Agent	Drug/Intervention	Category
PCP	*CD4, ≤200/mm³*	AI
	TMP-SMX 1 DS/d, 1 SS/d, 3 DS/wk	AI
	Dapsone	AI
	Dapsone + pyrimethamine + leucovorin	AI
	Aerosolized pentamidine	AI
	Alternative regimens: parenteral pentamidine, Fansidar, clindamycin + primaquine, atovaquone trimetrexate—for consideration in unusual circumstances	CIII
	Isolation from patient with PCP—not recommended	CIII
Toxoplasmosis	*CD4, ≤100/mm³ and positive IgG serology*	AII
	TMP-SMX	AII
	Dapsone + pyrimethamine + leucovorin	AI
	Alternatives: Dapsone, pyrimethamine, azithromycin, clarithromycin; atovaquone—not recommended	DII
	Seronegative 1 HIV infection	
	Avoid undercooked meat, cat litter box, keep pet cat inside and avoid strays	BIII
Cryptosporidosis	*All patients*	
	Avoid contact with human and animal feces; avoid purchasing dog or cat <6 mo old, strays or pets with diarrhea	BIII
	Outbreaks linked to municipal water:	
	Boil water	AI
	Use submicron filter or bottled water	CIII
Tuberculosis	*All patients*	
	Avoid high risk activities or occupations i.e., health care facilities, correctional institutions, shelters, etc.	BIII
	Positive PPD	AI
	No evidence active disease—INH +	AI
	Pyridoxine	BIII
	INH prophylaxis by DOT	BIII
	Alternate to INH: Rifampin	BIII
		CIII

	Close contact with tuberculosis—INH prophylaxis	AII
	PPD negative—annual PPD testing	BIII
	Anergy testing—not recommended	CIII
	PPD negative and high risk—not recommended	CIII
	Chronic suppressive therapy after completion of recommended regimen—not recommended	EII
	Pregnancy + POS PPD—INH after 1st trimester	AII
MAC	*CD4 cell count <75 (or 50)/mm*^{3}	
	Rifabutin prophylaxis	BII
	Clarithromycin	AI
	Azithromycin prophylaxis	AI
Bacterial infections respiratory tract	*All patients*	AII
	S. pneumoniae—pneumococcoal vaccine	AII
	Bacterial infections of respiratory tract TMP-SMX—given daily	AII
	Clarithromycin or azithromycin	BII
	H. influenzae vaccine—not recommended	DIII
	Neutropenia G-CSF or GM-CSF: not recommended	AII
Bacterial enteric infection	*All patients*	BIII
	Salmonella—avoid raw or undercooked eggs	
	Listerosis—avoid soft cheese and ready-to-eat food (hot dogs, cold cuts, etc.) or re-heat	CIII
	Pets—avoid pets <6 mo old & pets with diarrhea	BIII
	Avoid contact with reptiles	BIII
	Travel—Avoid potentially contaminated food and water	AII
	Prophylactic antibiotics depending on CD4 count and region	CIII
	Fluoroquinolone prophylaxis	BIII
Bartonella	*All patients,* esp. those with low CD4 counts	
	Avoid cat ownership	CIII
	or purchase cat >1 yr & healthy	BII
	Culture pet cat—not recommended	DII
Candidiasis	*Advanced HIV disease*	
	Fluconazole prophylaxis—not recommended	DII
Cryptococcosis	*CD4 count <50/mm*^{3}	
	Routine cryptococcal antigen testing—not recommended	CI
	Fluconazole prophylaxis—not recommended (but it is effective—BI)	DII

Table 16. ***(continued)***

Agent	Drug/Intervention	Category
Histoplasmosis	*All patients*	
	Avoid risk in endemic areas—cleaning chicken coops, exploring caves, etc.	CIII
	Routine histoplasmin skin test—not recommended	EII
	Chemoprophylaxis—not recommended	
Coccidioidomycosis	*All patients*	
	Avoid risk in endemic areas	CIII
	Chemoprophylaxis—no data	
	Routine skin test—no data	
Cytomegalovirus	*Patients with low risk*—CMV serology	BIII
	Seronegative patients—transfusion with CMV negative or leukocyte reduced cellular products	BIII
	Advanced HIV infection (CD4 <50/mm^3)	
	Oral ganciclovir—no recommendation	CII
	Acyclovir—not recommended	EII
	Regular funduscopic exam	CIII
Herpes simplex	*All patients*	
	Use of condoms	AII
	Avoid sex when lesions are active	AII
	Prophylaxis for initial episode—not recommended	DIII
Varicella zoster	*Susceptible (seronegative) pts.*	
	Avoid exposure to chicken pox and shingles	AII
	Close contact with case—Zoster immune globulin	AI
Human papilloma Virus	*All patients*	
	Use of condoms	AII
	HPV-associated cancer in women	
	Pap smear twice the first year and then annually if negative	AII
	Pap smear abnormal—Pap smear q 6 mo	BII
	Pap smear showing inflammation with reaction squamous cellular changes—repeat Pap smear within 3 mo	BIII
	Pap smear showing atypical changes—annual Pap smear	BIII
	Pap smear showing low grade SIL—repeat Pap smear within 3 mo, then: refer for colposcopy	BIII
	or repeat Pap smear q 3–6 mo	BIII
	Pap smear showing high grade SIL—refer for colposcopy	AI

Table 17. Recommendations for Opportunistic Infection Prophylaxis During Pregnancy

P. carinii:	Standard guidelines should be followed Some may choose to delay prophylaxis until after the first trimester Should use the full dose of TMP-SMX (1 DS/day) due to the increased blood volume
S. pneumoniae:	Pneumovax may be given safely in pregnancy
Toxoplasmosis:	Delay prophylaxis with pyrimethamine-containing regimens due to risk associated with this drug and the low probability of toxoplasmosis TMP-SMX prophylaxis is acceptable
M. avium:	Standard guidelines should be followed, but some may wish to defer or interrupt prophylaxis during the first trimester Experience with azithromycin, clarithromycin, and rifabutin are limited; azithromycin has proven safe in annual pregnancy studies; clarithromycin includes a warning that benefit must outrank the risk
Tuberculosis:	Standard treatment for positive PPD The routine chest x-ray should be delayed until after the first trimester INH treatment should include pyridoxine Rifampin or rifabutin should be used with caution
Varicella-zoster:	Zoster immune globulin is not contraindicated in pregnancy and should be given to a susceptible pregnant woman after exposure
Fungal infection:	Fluconazole has been associated with fetal deaths and fetal abnormalities in animal studies

Table 18. Recommendations for Vaccines in HIV-Infected Patients[a]

Vaccine	Indication	Regimen (Cost[b])	Comment
Routine vaccinations			
Pneumococcal vaccine	All HIV patients	0.5 mL IM ($11.90)	Risk of *S. pneumoniae* infection is increased 100-fold. Antigenic response is best when CD4 count is >200
Influenza vaccine	All HIV patients in Oct–Dec	0.5 mL IM ($4.37)	Risk of influenza is not clearly increased, but prevention may avoid expensive and complicated diagnostic evaluation of flu-like complaints. Vaccination may increase HIV viral burden, but significance is unknown and natural infection may increase it more.
Hepatitis B vaccine	See comments	3 IM doses at 0, 1, and 6 mo. Recombivax: 10 μg. Engerix: 20 μg ($55.78/dose or about $165 for the series)	Indications: Seronegative IDU, sexually active gay men, heterosexual men and women with STD or >1 sex partner in past 6 mo and household or sex contacts of HBsAg carriers Screening test is anti-HBc Risk of becoming HBsAg carrier is increased with HIV infection CDC recommends measurement of antibody response in HIV infected patients at 1–6 months after 3rd dose; non-responders should receive 1–3 boosters

Travel-associated vaccines			
Oral polio	Contraindicated	—	Live vaccine; eIPV preferred If inadvertently given to household contact, contact should be avoided for one month
Inactivated polio (eIPV)	Travel to developing countries for those without prior immunization	0.5 mL subcutaneously ($14.00)	Preferred for HIV-infected persons and close contracts Polio has beem eliminated from Western hemisphere
Yellow fever	Contraindicated		Live vaccine. With travel to endemic area advise patient of risk, instruct in control of mosquito exposure and provide vaccination waiver letter
Japanese B. encephalitis	Travel >1 mo to epidemic area	1 mL subcutaneously ×3 at days 0, 7, and 30 ($200)	Expensive and side effects (not unique to HIV-infected persons)
Typhoid (ViCSP) Typhoid inactivated vaccine	Travel to risk area (Latin America, Asia, Africa) (Same)	0.5 mL intramuscularly × 1. ($32.44) 0.25 ml subcutaneously × 2 separated by 1 month ($10.16/20 doses)	The live attenuated Ty21a vaccine (Vivotif) is contraindicated. ViCSP is the new Vi capsular polysaccharide vaccine which is no more effective than the parenteral inactivated vaccine, but causes fewer side effects and requires only one dose.
Hepatitis A	Travel to developing countries Gay men, injection drug users	1 mL adult formulation intramuscularly ×1 ≥ 14 days prior	Havrix was FDA approved in 1995 and may be used in place of immune globulin. Serologic tests show 30% of adults are protected by prior infection
Cholera vaccine	Not recommended	0.5 mL SC ×2 ≥ 1 wk apart ($8.38/1.5 ml)	This vaccine is no longer recommended nor required.

Table 18. *(continued)*

Vaccine	Indication	Regimen (Cost[b])	Comment
Other Vaccines			
Haemophilus influenzae type B	Not recommended	0.5 mg IM $\times 1$ ($20.46/dose)	Not recommended because most infections with *H. influenzae* in HIV-infected persons involve non-typable strains (JAMA 1992;268: 3350)
Tetanus-diphtheria (Td) vaccine	All adults—booster q 10 yrs	0.5 mg IM q 10 yrs ($2.40)	HIV infection is not a contraindication
Measles, mumps, rubella (MMR) vaccine	Contraindicated	—	Live virus vaccine; one report of a serious reaction (MMWR 1995;43: 959)
Varicella-zoster vaccine	Contraindicated in patients	—	Live virus vaccine; over 90% of adults have serologic evidence of varicella infection; if HIV-infected person is seronegative—avoid contact with chicken pox & zoster, and vaccinate susceptible close contacts

a

b

5—Antiretroviral Therapy

Three nearly simultaneous developments revolutionized HIV care during the period of 1995–97. First, simultaneous reports from the University of Alabama and the Aron Diamond Center showed that HIV replicated at a rate that produced 10 billion virions daily throughout most of the course of the disease (Nature 1995;373:117 and 223). This work clearly identified HIV as the primary target of any therapeutic attack. In early 1996 there was the introduction of quantitative plasma HIV RNA as a method to determine prognosis and response to therapy. This test quickly became embraced as a standard assay for routine monitoring. The third development was in therapeutics. After nearly a decade of nucleoside analogues, there was the introduction of nonnucleoside RT inhibitors (nevirapine, delavirdine) and protease inhibitors (saquinavir, indinavir, ritonavir, and nelfinavir). These newer drugs represent the most active agents available, but they also introduced new complexities in care due to the complexity of regimens, high rates of toxicity, and major concerns about resistance. This summary of antiretroviral therapy is divided into the following topics:

Table 19: Summary of Antiretroviral drugs

Recommendations for antiretroviral therapy (Johns Hopkins HIV Care Service)

Recommendations for prevention of perinatal transmission (CDC)

Recommendations for prevention of transmission in health care workers

Drug Summary

Antiretroviral Treatment of HIV-Infected Patients

I. Indications for Antiretroviral Therapy (Table 20)

- Acute HIV infection or within 6 months of seroconversion
- Decision based on viral burden and CD4 count <500/mm^3 *or* viral burden >10,000 copies/mL.

Table 19. Summary of Antiretroviral Drugs

Agent	Usual Regimen	Comment
Nucleoside Analogues (NRTIs) (See Table 22)		
• Zidovudine (Retrovir, AZT, ZDV)	300 mg bid or 200 mg tid	
• Didanosine (Videx, ddI)	200 mg bid	Empty stomach
• Zalcitabine (HIVID, ddC)	0.75 mg tid	
• Stavudine (Zerit, d4T)	40 mg bid	
• Lamivudine (Epivir, 3TC)	150 mg bid	
Protease Inhibitors (PIs) (See Table 23)		
• Saquinavir (Invirase)	600 mg tid	High fat meal
• Ritonavir (Norvir)	600 mg bid	Escalating dose refrigerate;
• Indinavir (Crixivan)	800 mg q 8h	Empty stomach or light meal; >2 liters fluid/d
• Nelfinavir (Viracept)	750 mg tid	With meals
Non-Nucleoside RT Inhibitor (NNRTIs)		
• Nevirapine (Viramune)	200 mg bid	200 mg qd, then 200 mg bid
• Delavirdine (Rescriptor)	400 mg bid	

Table 20. Indications for Antiretroviral Therapy

CD4 (/mm^3)	Viral Burden (copies/mL)	Treatment
>500	<10,000	Observe
>500	>10,000	Offer treatment*
<500	(Any value)	Offer treatment*

* The strength of the recommendation to treat depends on patient acceptance of a complex regimen and prognosis as determined by CD4 count and viral burden.

II. Initial Regimen

A. PREFERRED. Two nucleoside RT inhibitors (NRTIs) and a protease inhibitor (PI)*

2 NRTIs (no order)	PI (no order)
AZT + 3TC or	Nelfinavir or
AZT + ddI or	Indinavir or
AZT + ddC or	Ritonavir or
d4T + 3TC or	
d4T + ddI	

Advantage. Optimal regimens for maximal reduction in viral burden for the greatest duration.

Disadvantage. Medically complex in terms of need for compliance, "pill burden," and potential toxicity. Evolution of resistance with these regimens is less likely than with alternative treatments, but if resistance occurs, this may severely limit future options for protease inhibitors and nucleosides.

B. ALTERNATIVE. Two nucleoside RT inhibitors and nevirapine—nevirapine plus: AZT + 3TC, AZT + ddI, AZT + ddC, d4T + 3TC, or d4T + ddI

Advantage. These regimens are generally well tolerated and somewhat simplified compared with most regimens that include protease inhibitors. This treatment preserves the option for likely success with protease-inhibitor regimens since there is no cross-resistance.

Disadvantage. Clinical trials have not shown advantages in terms of clinical outcome, and viral burden data is less convincing in terms of the frequency of achieving the goal of no detectable virus.

---

* Preferred treatment requires assiduous attention to compliance with a complex medical regimen lasting several years. This is preferred because there are controlled trials showing substantial benefit in terms of clinical outcome (time to an AIDS-defining diagnosis or death) and surrogate marker response (CD4 count increase and reduction in viral burden). These trials show persistent benefit for >1 year in a modest number of participants.

C. SECOND ALTERNATIVE FOR SELECTED PATIENTS. Two nucleoside RT inhibitors—AZT + 3TC, AZT + ddI, AZT + ddC, d4T + 3TC, or d4T + ddI

Advantage. Substantial data from clinical trials showing benefit in terms of clinical outcome and surrogate marker outcome. These regimens are generally relatively simple and well tolerated.

Disadvantage. Suboptimal results in major outcome objective since the number that achieve no detectable virus is a minority and the duration of this effect, when achieved, is usually limited. The double-nucleoside regimens also constitute exposure to these drugs so that use of the "preferred regimen" in the future may be compromised due to resistance or toxicity.

D. CONTRAINDICATED. Monotherapy with any antiretroviral drug or any of the following combinations: AZT + d4T, ddI + ddC, or d4T + ddC

Rationale. (1) Clinical trials show substantial inferiority of single drug regimens in the number who achieve no detectable virus and the duration of response regimens; (2) clinical trials show rapid development of high-level resistance plus clinical progression—monotherapy with 3TC, nevirapine, or any protease inhibitor; (3) possible in vitro and in vivo antagonism—AZT + d4T, and (4) lack of any supporting clinical trials plus overlapping toxicity—ddI + ddC and d4T + ddC.

III. When to Change Therapy

A. THERAPEUTIC FAILURE

1. *No detectable virus using a viral burden assay with a threshold of <500 copies/mL.* This is the goal and the usual expectation of the preferred regimens. The maximum antiviral effect is achieved at 3–6 months so that failure to show no detectable virus at that time constitutes failure. The failure to decrease viral burden >1 log at 4 weeks after initiating treatment usually predicts treatment failure. There may need to be a distinction between partial or incomplete response and patients who have no response or respond and then fail. Other presumably important variables are the CD4 strata and viral burden. The experience with these variables is too limited to give specific guidance.
2. *Modified and other goals*

a. Significant decrease in viral load, because "no detectable virus" is deemed unrealistic.
b. CD4 count increase: There is sometimes a paradoxical decrease in both viral burden and CD4 count. This may be due to laboratory error, SI vs. non-SI strains of HIV, and other causes of CD4 lymphopenia; most commonly it is explained by a delayed CD4 response. The viral burden should take precedence in therapeutic monitoring.
c. HIV-related complications: These may indicate therapeutic failure, or may reflect conditions that were incubating at the time the new regimen was initiated.

B. TOXICITY OF REGIMEN OR NEED FOR DRUGS THAT PRECLUDE CONTINUATION DUE TO INTERACTIONS (E.G., ACTIVE TUBERCULOSIS)

C. NONACCEPTANCE OR NONCOMPLIANCE

D. AVAILABILITY OF A NEW REGIMEN THAT HAS BENEFICIAL FEATURES IN TERMS OF ANTIVIRAL ACTIVITY, TOLERANCE, OR TOXICITY

IV. What to Change to

A. FAILURE OF REGIMEN. There needs to be ≥2 new antiretroviral agents and preferably a completely new 3-4 drug regimen.

1. *Failed regimen: Two nucleosides and a protease inhibitor*
   New regimen
   a. Two new nucleosides plus either nevirapine or a protease inhibitor selected on the basis of predicted sensitivity. Examples of appropriate combinations: AZT + 3TC, AZT + ddI, AZT + ddC, d4T + 3TC, or d4T + ddI *plus* either nevirapine or a new protease inhibitor.

      Protease inhibitor changes*

      Nelfinavir → Ritonavir or indinavir or combination treatment

      Ritonavir → Nelfinavir (?) or combination treatment*

      Indinavir → Nelfinavir (?) or combination treatment*

      Saquinavir → Nelfinavir or ritonavir or indinavir or combination treatment*
   b. Combination treatment with two protease inhibitors or a protease inhibitor plus nevirapine, usually with one or more nucleoside analogues (see Table 24). Experience in

the use of these combinations is limited, but examples of combinations that appear promising based on preliminary data from clinical trials phase-2 pharmacology studies or from theoretical advantages.

*Combination regimens (See Table 24)
Ritonavir + saquinavir ± or two nucleosides
Nevirapine + indinavir ± 1 or 2 nucleosides
Nevirapine + ritonavir ± 1 or 2 nucleosides
Nelfinavir + saquinavir ± 1 or 2 nucleosides
Nelfinavir + ritonavir ± 1 or 2 nucleosides
Nelfinavir + saquinavir ± 1 or 2 nucleosides

2. *Failed regimen: Two nucleosides + nevirapine*

   New regimen: Two nucleosides including at least one new nucleoside plus a protease inhibitor.

   Examples of appropriate combinations: AZT + 3TC, AZT + ddI, AZT + ddC, d4T + 3TC, or d4T + ddI *plus* either ritonavir, or nelfinavir.
3. *Failed regimen: Two nucleoside analogues*

   New regimen: Two new nucleosides a protease inhibitor or nevirapine.

   Examples of appropriate combinations: AZT + 3TC, AZT + ddI, AZT + ddC, d4T + 3TC, or d4T + ddI plus either nevirapine, ritonavir, nelfinavir, or indinavir.

B. TOXICITY OR INTOLERANCE. Drug substitution using two nucleosides and a protease inhibitor. There is no need for two new agents if therapeutic goals were achieved.

C. NONCOMPLIANCE. Discontinue treatment or substitute a simplified regimen such as 2 nucleosides + nevirapine, 2 nucleosides.

Recommendations of the U.S. Public Health Service Task Force on the Use of Zidovudine (AZT) to Reduce Perinatal Transmission of HIV (MMWR 1994;43(RR-11):1–20) and Testing of Pregnant Women (MMWR 1995;44(RR-7):1–14). [Recommendations are based on ACTG 076], which showed that AZT reduced the rate of perinatal transmission from 28% to 8% (N Engl J Med 1994;331:1173). A subsequent report showed that the protective effect of AZT was not dependent on a detectable antiviral effect in the mother (N Engl J Med 1996;335:1621)).

Current guidelines are (1) Routine HIV counseling and voluntary testing for all pregnant women and (2) pregnant women with HIV infection should be offered AZT therapy in the regimen employed in ACTG 076:

Before delivery: AZT (100 mg 5×/day) initiated at 14–34 weeks of gestation and continued to onset of labor.
During labor: IV AZT (loading infusion of 2 mg/kg IV for one hr followed by continuous infusion 1 mg/kg per hr until delivery)
Infant: AZT for the newborn (AZT syrup at 2 mg/kg every 6 hrs) for the first 6 weeks of life beginning 8–12 hrs after birth.

Note. These recommendations are now somewhat antiquated by recommendations for HIV infection in the mother, which should take precedence. In general, pregnant women should receive AZT to prevent perinatal transmission since this is the only drug with established merit. However, most pregnant women will merit more aggressive treatment based on the recommendations summarized above despite the lack of studies establishing safely in pregnancy for nearly all antiretroviral agents (Table 20).

Postexposure Prophylaxis for Health Care Workers

A total of 23 needlestick studies in health care workers showed HIV transmission in 20 of 6135 (0.33%) exposed to an HIV-infected source (Ann Intern Med 1990;113:740). With mucosal surface exposure there was one transmission in 1143 exposures (0.09), and there were no transmissions in 2712 skin exposures. As of June 1996, there were a total of 49 health care workers in the US who had occupationally acquired HIV infection as indicated by seroconversion in the context of an exposure to an HIV-infected source. There are an additional 102 health care workers who have possible occupationally acquired HIV; these health care workers did not have seroconversion in the context of an exposure. Of the 49 confirmed cases: (1) The major occupations were nurses and laboratory technicians. (2) All transmissions involved blood or bloody body fluid except for three involving lab workers exposed to HIV viral cultures. (3) To date there are no confirmed seroconversions in surgeons and no seroconversions with exposures to suture needles.

A case-control study of needlestick injuries from an HIV-infected source by the CDC included 37 cases who seroconverted and 739 controls (MMWR 1996;45:468). This showed that risks for seroconversion included: (1) deep injury; (2) visible blood on the device; (3) needle placement in a vein or artery, and (4) a source with late-stage HIV infection (presumably reflecting high viral load). There was also evidence that AZT prophylaxis was associated with a 79% reduction in transmission rates. On the basis of this experience, revised guidelines recommending more aggressive antiretroviral therapy were published in June 1996 (MMWR 1996;45:468) (see Table 21).

Comments regarding recommendations:

- **Drug selection:** The only drug with established merit for reducing HIV transmission with needlestick injuries is AZT (Retrovir). The rationale for recommending AZT plus 3TC (lamivudine) is based on the greater antiretroviral activity of this combination when given to patients with established infection. The addition of a protease inhibitor reflects greater antiviral potency with the recommendation for high-risk injuries and settings in which resistance to AZT and/or 3TC is anticipated based on the treatment regimen of the source. The preference for indinavir reflects the options at the time of the recommendations (March 1996): saquinavir is poorly absorbed and ritonavir is poorly tolerated. Nelfinavir has subsequently been FDA approved (3/14/97) and represents a rational alternative with the possible advantage of sparse side effects. Nevirapine is another option; the major disadvantage is the high rate of rash reactions (18%) and rare cases of Stevens-Johnson syndrome.
- **Side effects:** The major side effects of AZT are GI intolerance, headache, and fatigue (Ann Intern Med 1993;118:913). Stavudine (d4T) is an appropriate alternative for those who do not tolerate AZT, although AZT is the only drug with established efficacy. There are few side effects with 3TC. The major risks with indinavir are GI intolerance (10%) and renal calculi (0.8% with treatment for 1 month). It is necessary for recipients of indinavir to take >48 oz of fluid daily to reduce the probability of renal calculi.

Table 21. Provisional Public Health Service Recommendations for Chemoprophylaxis After Occupational Exposure to HIV, by Type of Exposure and Source Material—1996

Type of Exposure	Source Material	Antiretroviral Prophylaxis[a]	Antiretroviral Regimen[b]
Percutaneous	Blood[c]		
	Highest risk	Recommend	ZDV plus 3TC plus IDV
	Increased risk	Recommended	ZDV plus 3TC, ± IDV
	No increased risk	Offer	ZDV plus 3TC
	Fluid containing visible blood, other potentially infectious fluid, or tissue	Offer	ZDV plus 3TC
	Other body fluid (e.g., urine)	Not offer	
Mucous membrane	Blood	Offer	ZDV plus 3TC, ±IDV
	Fluid containing visible blood, other potentially infectious fluid[d], or tissue	Offer	ZDV, ±3TC
	Other body fluid (e.g., urine)	Not offer	
Skin, increased risk	Blood	Offer	ZDV plus 3TC, ±IDV
	Fluid containing visible flood, other potentially infectious fluid[d], or tissue	Offer	ZDV, ±3TC
	Other body fluid (e.g., urine)	Not offer	

[a] Recommend postexposure prophylaxis (PEP); offer—indicates offering PEP; Not offer—PEP should not be offered
[b] ZDV = Retrovir or AZT (200 mg po tid or 300 mg po bid); 3TC (Lamivudine) (150 mg po bid), IDV = Indinavir (800 mg po q8h)
[c] Highest risk: Large volume inoculum and high HIV titer specimen
[d] Includes semen, vaginal secretions, and cerebrospinal, synovial, pleurisy, perineal, pericardial, and amniotic fluids. (Note that all seroconversions have involved blood or bloody body fluid or viral cultures in labs)

- **Pregnancy testing:** Some facilities require a pregnancy test prior to administration of AZT postexposure prophylaxis in female health care workers with childbearing potential. The relevance of this recommendation is enhanced by the NCI report of January 1997 that AZT in doses of 12–15× those recommended for patients are carcinogenic to the offspring of pregnant mice. Although there is no evidence of similar toxicity in patients, this is an important component of the informed choice. There is minimal information about the safety of indinavir and 3TC during pregnancy.
- **Timing:** Prophylaxis should be initiated as rapidly as possible after exposure, preferably within 1–2 hours. Animal studies show no benefit when treatment is delayed 24–36 hours (JID 1993;168:1490; N Engl J Med 1995;332:444); nevertheless, the CDC recommends prophylaxis with a delay of up to 1–2 weeks with high-risk exposures. The Hopkins program includes a 72-hour "starter pack" to promote early prophylaxis when the health care worker is undecided. There is also a service to deliver initial doses to the operating room to prevent the need to break scrub.
- **Monitoring:** HIV serology is performed at baseline, 6 wks, 12 wks, and 6 months. We are aware of only one HCW who seroconverted at >6 months after occupational exposure. For patients who receive postexposure prophylaxis, the drug toxicity monitoring should include a CBC and hepatic and renal function tests at baseline and at 2 weeks after treatment is initiated.
- **Reporting:** HCWs who receive postexposure prophylaxis are encouraged to report experiences to an anonymous registry 888-737-4448.

AGENTS

NUCLEOSIDE ANALOGUES

AZT (Zidovudine) *Trade name:* Retrovir (Glaxo-Wellcome)

Dose regimens

Usual regimen: 200 mg po tid or 300 mg bid
Minimum effective dose: 100 mg po tid
HIV-associated dementia: 1000–1200 mg/day

Table 22. Nucleoside Analogues

Trade Name	Zidovudine (AZT, ZDV) Retrovir	Didanosine (ddI) Videx	Zalcitabine (ddC) HIVID	Stavudine (d4T) Zerit	Lamivudine (3TC) Epivir
How supplied	100 and 300 mg tabs IV vials—10 mg/ml	25, 50, 100, and 150 mg tabs 100, 167, and 250 mg powder packets	0.375 and 0.75 mg tabs	15, 20, 30, and 40 mg caps	150 mg tabs
Usual dose	200 mg tid or 300 mg bid	Tablets >60 kg: 200 mg bid <60 kg: 125 mg bid	0.75 mg tid	>60 kg: 40 mg bid <60 kg: 30 mg bid	150 mg bid
Minimum effective dose	300 mg/d	200 mg/d (powder)	Not studied	Not studied	Not studied
Oral bioavailability	60%	Tablet: 40% Powder: 30%	85%	86%	86%
Serum half-life	1.1 hour	1.6 hour	1.2 hour	1.0 hour	3–6 hours
Intracellular half-life	3 hours	12 hours	3 hours	3.5 hours	12 hours
CNS penetration (% serum levels)	60%	20%	20%	30–40%	10%
Elimination	Metabolized to AZT glucuronide (GAZT) Renal extraction GAZT	Renal excretion—50%	Renal excretion—70%	Renal excretion—50% unchanged	Renal excretion
Major toxicity	Bone marrow suppression: Anemia and/or neutropenia Subjective complaints: GI intolerance, headache, insomnia, asthenia	Pancreatitis Peripheral neuropathy	Peripheral neuropathy Stomatitis	Peripheral neuropathy	(Minimal toxicity)
Mutations conferring resistance (codon)	41[a], 67, 70[a], 215[a], 219	65, 69, 74, 75, 184	65, 69, 74, 75, 184, 215	41, 50, 70, 75	65, 184[a]

[a] Mutations considered most clinically significant.

Table 23. Protease Inhibitors

	Saquinavir	Ritonavir	Indinavir	Nelfinavir
Trade name	Invirase	Norvir	Crixivan	Viracept
Supplier	Hoffman-LaRoche	Abbott	Merck	Agouron
Form	200 mg caps	100 mg caps	200, 400 mg caps	250 mg caps[a]
Usual dose	600 mg tid*	600 mg bid[a]	800 mg q8h	750 mg tid
Bioavailability (Recommendations)	hard capsule: 4% soft capsule: 12% (with high-fat meal)	70–90% (taken with food) Refrigerate	60–70% (empty stomach)	20–80% (with food)
Serum half-life	1–2 hrs	3–4 hrs	1.5–2 hrs	3.5–5 hrs
CNS penetration	Poor	Poor	Moderate (?)	Moderate
Elimination	Biliary metabolism P450 cytochrome 3A	Biliary metabolism P450 cytochrome 3A, 2D, 2C	Biliary metabolism P450 cytochrome 3A	Biliary metabolism P450 cytochrome 3A
Side effects	GI intolerance (5%) Headache	GI intolerance (20–40%) Paresthias—circumoral and extremities 10% Taste perversion 10% Lab Triglycerides ↑ (60%) transaminase ↑ (10–15%)	GI intolerance (10–15%) Nephrolithiasis (5–10%) Lab: ↑ indirect bilirubin	Diarrhea (2–10%)

Drug interactions	Drugs to increase saquinavir levels: Ritonavir, Ketoconazole Nelfinavir, grapefruit juice Contraindicated drugs: Terfenadine, astemizole, cisapride, rifampin	Potent inhibition of P450 enzymes Contraindicated drugs[b]	Inhibition of P450 enzymes (less than ritonavir) Contraindicated drugs: Terfenadine, astemizole, cisapride, rifampin, midazolam, triazolam	Inhbition of P450 enzymes (less than ritonavir) Contraindicated drugs: Terfenadine, astemizole, cisapride midazolam, trazolam rifampin
Codon mutations associated with resistance, indicates most signifcant	10, 48, 63, 71, 84, (90)	20, (36), 46, (54), 63, 71, (82), 84, 90	(10), 20, 24, 36, (46), 54, (63), 66, 71, (82), 84, 90	(30), (71), 77, 84

[a] Dose escalation for Ritonavir: Day 1–2: 300 mg bid; day 6–13: 500 mg bidl; day ≥14: 600 mg bid. Combination treatment regimen with Saquinavir (400 mg po bid) plus Ritonavir (400–600 mg po bid).

[b] Drugs contraindicated for concurrent use with Ritonavir: alprazolam (Xanax), amioderone (Cordarone), astemizole (Hismanal), bepridil (Vascor), bupropion (Wellbutrin), cisapride (Propulsid), clorazepate (Tranxene), clozapine (Clozanl), diazepam (Valium), encainide (Enkaid), ergot alkaloids, estazolam (ProSom), flecainide (Tambocor), flurazepam (Dalmane), meperidine (Demerol), midazolam (Versed), pimozide, piroxicam (Feldene), propoxyphene (Darvon), propofenone (Rythmol), quinidine, rifabutin (Mycobutin), terfenadine (Seldane), triazolam (Halcion), zolpidem (Ambien). Decreased levels of clarithromycin (Biaxin), ethinyl estradiol (contraceptives), theophylline, sulfamethoxazole and Retrovir (AZT).

Table 24. Drug Interactions

	Saquinavir	Ritonavir	Indinavir	Nelfinavir	Nevirapine	Delavirdine
Saquinavir (SQV)	X	Levels: SQV ↑ 20×; RIT no effect Dose: SQV 400 mg bid + RIT 400–600 mg bid	Levels: SQV ↑ 4–7×; IND no effect Dose: No data	Levels: SQV ↑ 3–5×, NFV no effect Dose: No data	Levels: SQV ↓ 25% Avoid use	Levels: SQV ↑ 5× Dose: Standard
Ritonavir (RTV)	Levels: RIT no effect; SQV ↑ 10× Dose: SQV 400 mg bid + RTV 400–600 mg bid	X	No data	Levels: RTV no effect; NFV ↑ 2× Dose: No data	Levels: RTV no effect Dose: Standard	Levels: RTV no effect Dose: Standard
Indinavir (IND)	Levels: IND no effect; SQV ↑ 4–7× Dose: No data	No data	X	Levels: IND ↑ 50%; NFV ↑ 2.5× Dose: No data	Levels: IND ↓ 10–30% Dose: IND 1000 mg tid	Levels: IND ↑ 2× Dose: IND 600 mg q 8 h
Nelfinavir (NFV)	Levels: NFV no effect; SQV ↑ 3× Dose: Standard	Levels: NFV ↑ 2×; RTV no effect Dose: No data	Levels: NFV ↑ 80%; IND ↑ 50% Dose: No data	X	Levels: NFV ↓ Dose: NFV 1000 mg tid (?)	No data
Nevirapine (NVP)	Levels: SQV ↓ Avoid use	Levels: RTV no effect Dose: Standard	Levels: NVP ↑ 2×; IND ↓ 10–30% Dose: IND 1000 mg tid	No data	X	No data
Delavirdine (DVD)	Levels: SQV ↑ 5× Dose: Standard	Levels: RTV levels unchanged Dose: Standard	Levels: IND ↑ 2× Dose: IND 600 mg tid	No data	No data	X

Pregnancy: 100 mg 5×/day; delivery—2 mg/kg/hr × 1 hr, then 1 mg/kg/hr until delivery; infant received 2 mg/kg po q 6 h × 6 wks (MMWR 1994;43:RR-1:1)

Postexposure in health care workers: 200 mg po tid or 300 mg po bid × 4 weeks (MMWR 1995;44:929)

Renal failure: No clear guidelines; some use half-dose with creatinine clearance <10 mL/min

Forms available: 100 mg and 300 mg tabs; IV vials—10 mg/mL; 20 mL

Cost: $1.55/100 mg tab; $3.98/300 mg tab

Financial assistance: 800-722-9294

Pharmacology: Absorption—60%; T½ serum—1.1 hr; T½ serum with renal failure—1.4 hr; T½ intracellular—3 hr; CNS penetration—60%; elimination—metabolized to AZT glucuronide which is renally excreted as G-AZT.

Note: AZT has superior CNS penetration compared with alternative nucleoside analogues and protease inhibitors. This may be an important factor in selection of drugs used in combination.

Monitoring: CBC q 3 mo; LFTs q 3–6 mo

Note: Nearly all patients develop clinically inconsequential macrocytosis within 4 weeks of initiating AZT. The lack of macrocytosis should raise concern about compliance.

Side effects

Major:

1. *Subjective complaints* with headache, malaise, GI intolerance, insomnia, and/or asthenia—dose related and may resolve with continued treatment.
2. *Marrow suppression* with anemia and/or neutropenia—frequency and severity related to dose, duration, and stage. Management: Reduce dose or discontinue with Hgb ≤7.5 g/dL or absolute neutrophile count (ANC) <75–1000/mm^3; alternative is co-administration of G-CSF or EPO.

Minor or infrequent: *Myopathy* with increased CPK; *hepatitis* with increased transaminase levels; *lactic acidosis* with steatosis and fulminant hepatic failure (obese women and patients with liver disease appear to be at risk; *cardiomyopathy* with reduced LV function by ECHO; *fingernail discoloration* (common and not important)

Drug interactions: Concurrent use with ganciclovir and other marrow-suppressing agents is contraindicated. Use with caution and monitor CBC carefully with dapsone, TMP-SMX, flucytosine, interferon, sulfadiazine, and amphotericin. There is antagonism in vitro and possibly in vivo when used in combination with d4T (stavudine).

Pregnancy: The National Cancer Institute reported in January 1997 that administration of AZT in doses 12–15× those used in patients proved carcinogenic to the offspring of pregnant mice. A second study by Glaxo-Wellcome using doses equivalent to those used in patients showed no carcinogenic potential in pregnant mice. The NIH subsequently convened a panel to review these data. The unanimous conclusion was that the established benefits of AZT for preventing perinatal transmission outweigh the hypothetical risk. Nevertheless, the pregnant patient or patient of childbearing potential should be aware of this issue.

ddI (Didanosine) *Trade name:* Videx (Bristol-Meyers-Squibb)

Dose regimens

Standard dose:

	Tablet[a]	Powder
≥60 kg	200 mg po bid	250 mg po bid
<60 kg	125 mg po bid	167 mg po bid

[a] Tabs must be chewed thoroughly or crushed and dissolved in water.

Minimum effective dose: 200 mg/day (powder)

Renal failure: Guidelines are not available; main concern is Na^+ (11.5 mEq/tab) and Mg^{++} (15.7 mEq/tab). With dialysis, reduce dose to one fourth the standard dose

Forms: Tabs of 25, 50, 100, and 150 mg (mandarin orange flavored). Powder packets of 100, 167, and 250 mg

Cost: $1.53/100 mg tab

Financial assistance: 800-272-4878

***Indications* (Based on ACTG 116/117 and 175):** Patients with CD4 counts and <500/mm³ treated with ddI monotherapy (AZT experienced or AZT naive) show a significant reduction in rates of disease progression based on clinical endpoints compared with AZT monotherapy. AZT plus ddI also show superior results compared with AZT alone. A concern is incomplete viral suppression or limited duration of viral suppression as determined by sequential viral burden assays. Superior antiviral activity is noted when ddI is combined with a second nucleoside analogue and a protease inhibitor.

Pharmacology

Oral absorption—30 to 40%; T1/2 serum—1.6 hr; T1/2 intracellular—12 hr; CNS penetration—20%; elimination—renal

Monitoring: Amylase q 1–2 mo is sometimes advocated; most important is to warn patient of symptoms of pancreatitis and peripheral neuropathy.

Side effects

Major:

1. *Peripheral neuropathy* in 1–12% related to dose and duration. Management: discontinue ddI or reduce dose.
2. *Pancreatitis* in 1–9%; risk with history of pancreatitis, advanced HIV, alcoholism, and concurrent meds that cause pancreatitis. Management—reduce dose or discontinue if routine monitoring shows amylase is $\geq$1.5–2 $\times$ upper limit of normal.
3. *Gastrointestinal intolerance of formulation.* A new formulation that is smaller, easier to chew, and flavored with mandarin orange was introduced in June 1996. Other methods to improve tolerance are to dissolve tabs in ice water or apple juice, or try powder form. Alternatively (for 400 mg total daily dose), 200 mL water, 200 mL Maalox (double strength), or Mylanta (double strength) with one 4-g bottle of pediatric powder. A single dose is 25 mL. Remainder is kept refrigerated; this suspension is stable for 30 days.

Minor or infrequent: *Marrow suppression, hyperuricemia, hepatitis, rash,* Na^+ load (11.5 mEq/tab and 60 mEq/powder packet); Mg^{++} load (15.7 mEq/tab)

Drug interactions: Drugs requiring gastric acidity should be given 2 hr before or 2 hr after ddI—dapsone, ketoconazole, itraconazole, and tetracyclines. Drugs that cause pancreatitis should be used with caution—pentamidine, ethambutol, and alcohol. Drugs that cause peripheral neuropathy should be used with caution or avoided—cisplatin, ddC, d4T, disulfiram, ethionamide, INH, phenytoin, vincristine, hydralazine, metronidazole (long-term use only), and glutethimide.

ddC (Zalcitabine) *Trade name:* HIVID (Hoffman-LaRoche)

Dose regimen: 0.75 mg tid

Renal failure: Cr cl <50 ml/min—0.75 mg tid; 20–50 ml/min—0.75 mg bid; <10 ml/min—0.75 qd

Minimum effective dose: Not established

Form: 0.375 and 0.75 mg tabs

Cost: $2.29/0.75 mg tab

Financial assistance: 800-282-7780

***Indications* (Based on ACTG 155 and 175):** Patients with CD4 counts <500/mm^3 treated with ddC in combination with AZT (AZT-naive patients) had superior outcomes based on clinical criteria compared with monotherapy with AZT. A concern is the lack of complete or prolonged viral suppression. A preferrable regimen is ddC with another nucleoside analogue and a protease inhibitor.

Pharmacology

Oral bioavailability 85%; T½ serum—1.2–2 hr; T½ intracellular—3 hr; CNS penetration—20%; elimination: renal excretion—70%

Monitoring: Warn patient of symptoms of peripheral neuropathy

Side effects

Major: *Peripheral neuropathy* in 17–31%, related to dose and duration. Management: Discontinue; patients with mild symptoms or symptoms that have resolved may be treated with half dose.

Minor or infrequent: *Stomatitis, aphthous ulcers, pancreatitis, hepatitis*

Drug interactions: Drugs that cause peripheral neuropathy should be avoided or used with caution—ddI, d4T, cisplatin, disulfiram, ethionamide, INH, phenytoin, vincristine, glutethimide, gold, hydralazine, and metronidazole.

d4T (Stavudine) *Trade name:* Zerit (Bristol-Meyers-Squibb)

Dose Regimen: ≥60 kg—40 mg po bid; <60 kg—30 mg po bid

Renal failure: Cr clearance >50 mL/min—40 mg bid; 25–50 mL/min—20 mg bid; 10–25 mL/min—20 mg q 24 h

Forms: 15, 20, 30, and 40 mg caps

Cost: $3.46/15 mg cap; $3.60/20 mg cap; $3.60/30 mg cap; $3.88/40 mg cap

Financial assistance: 800-272-4878

Indications **(Based on BMS 019):** Patients with CD4 counts <500/mm^3 (± prior AZT therapy) treated with d4T monotherapy (Al 455-019) had rates of progression that were quite comparable to ddI monotherapy. There is limited experience with d4T in combination with other nucleoside analogues due to concerns about overlapping toxicity (peripheral neuropathy) with ddI and ddC, and in vitro antagonism with AZT. Nevertheless, trials with ddI plus AZT appeared to show good clinical results without excessive toxicity. It is now preferred to use d4T in triple-drug regimens with another nucleoside analogue and a protease inhibitor. Advantages of stavudine are the simplicity of the regimen (1 tab bid), good tolerance, and good CNS penetration.

Pharmacology

Oral bioavailability—86% (not influenced by food); T1/2 serum—1 hr; T1/2 intracellular—3.5 hr; CNS penetration—30%–40%; elimination: renal—50%

Monitoring: Warn patient of symptoms of peripheral neuropathy

Side effects

Major: *Peripheral neuropathy* in 15–21%, related to dose and duration

Infrequent or rare: *Pancreatitis, hepatitis, neutropenia*

Drug interactions: Drugs that cause peripheral neuropathy should be avoided or used with caution. Concurrent use with other nucleoside analogues that cause peripheral neuropathy (ddI and ddC) must be done with caution. There are conflicting data concerning in vitro antagonism with d4T plus AZT versus HIV, but a clinical trial supported the possibility of antagonism.

3TC (Lamivudine) *Trade name:* Epivir (Glaxo-Wellcome)

Dose regimen: 150 mg po bid

Renal failure: Cr clearance <50 mL/min—150 mg bid; 30–49 mL/min—150 mg qd; 15–29 mL/min—100 mg qd; 5–14 mL/min—50 mg qd; <5 mL/min—25 mg qd

Forms: 150 mg tabs and oral solution with 10 mg/mL

Cost: $3.11/150 mg tab

Financial assistance: 800-722-9294

***Indications* (Based on studies A3001, A3002, B3001, B3002, Caesar):** 3TC may be used in combination with AZT in patients (AZT experienced or AZT naive) with CD4 counts <500/mm^3 (N Engl J Med 1995;333:1662). Experience with 3TC in combination with other nucleoside analogues is limited. Short-term experience with AZT, 3TC, and indinavir showed viral burden decrease to <500/dL in 86% at 68 weeks; similar results were achieved with ritonavir.

Hepatitis B virus is inhibited by lamivudine (N Engl J Med 1995;333:1657); treatment of patients who were co-infected with HIV and HBV showed significant reduction in HBV DNA concentrations (Ann Intern Med 1996;125:705). Resistance by HBV is an anticipated problem.

Pharmacology

Oral bioavailability—86%; T½ serum—3–6 hr; T½ intracellular—12 hr; CNS penetration—10%; elimination—renal

Monitoring: CBC q 3 mo and LFTs q 3–6 mo (for AZT)

Side effects

Minor: *Headache, nausea, diarrhea, abdominal pain, and insomnia.*

PROTEASE INHIBITORS

Saquinavir *Trade name:* Invirase (Hoffman-LaRoche)

Dose: FDA approved dose is 600 mg (three 200-mg caps) tid taken within 2 hours of a fatty meal and given in combination with other antiretroviral agents. Antiviral effect is dose related: a daily dose of 7.2 g/day (36 tabs/day) (Ann Intern Med 1996;

124:108) produces a substantially greater decrease in viral burden and increase in CD4 cell response. Alternative methods that improve bioavailability are use of a new formulation ("soft gel capsule"); administration with a drug that inhibits cytochrome P450 such as ketoconazole (200 mg/day), indinavir, nelfinavir, delavirdine, or ritonavir; or co-administration with grapefruit juice.

Dose modification in renal failure or hepatic failure: None

Forms available: 200 mg caps

Cost: 200 mg cap $2.12

Financial assistance: 800-282-7780

Indications **(based on ACTG 229, V-13330, and HV 14259)** show: saquinavir plus AZT is superior to AZT alone and saquinavir plus ddC is superior to AZT plus ddC or ddC alone. Saquinavir plus ritonavir shows a 2–3 log decrease in plasma HIV RNA that is sustained for ≥52 weeks. Indicated for advanced HIV infection in combination with nucleoside analogues.

Pharmacology: Absorption—4% when taken with high-fat meal to promote absorption; T½ serum—1–2 hr; CNS penetration—poor; Elimination—96% biliary excretion via cytochrome p450, 1% in urine

Side effects: Dose-related GI intolerance with nausea, abdominal pain and diarrhea (4–6% with daily dose of 1.8 g/day); headache

Drug interactions: Rifampin reduces levels by 80% and rifabutin by 40%—concurrent use with either should be avoided. Other drugs that reduce Saquinavir levels are nevirapine, phenobarbital, phenytoin, dexamethasone, and carbamazepine. Clarithromycin should be used in place of rifabutin for MAC prophylaxis. Drugs that inhibit cytochrome p450 increase levels of Saquinavir, including ketoconazole (increase Saquinavir levels by 150%), itraconazole, and fluconazole; other antiretroviral agents that elevate Saquinavir levels by inhibition of cytochrome p450 3A are ritonavir (increases saquinavir levels >20 fold), indinavir (4–7 fold), and nelfinavir (3–5 fold). With nevirapine, there is induction of the p450 enzymes with reduction of saquinavir levels. Saquinavir may increase levels of terfenadine, astemizole, or cisapride causing ventricular arrhythmias; concurrent use is not recommended.

INDINAVIR *Trade name:* Crixivan (Merck Sharp and Dohme)

Form: 200 and 400 mg capsules

Cost: $2.50/400 mg cap

Patient assistance program: 800-850-3430

Clinical trials: Phase I/II trials show a dose-dependent antiviral effect; with 800 mg tid the mean decrease in viral burden was 1–1.5 logs in those receiving monotherapy and >2 logs with combination therapy using indinavir plus two nucleoside analogues. Indinavir + AZT + 3TC or ddI in patients with CD4 <500/mm^3 and viral burden >20,000/dL showed a mean CD4 count increase of 80–100/mm^3 and decreased viral burden to undetectable levels in 60–80% of patients for ≥68 weeks. Optimal results are achieved in patients who are treatment naive. A limited experience with nevirapine plus indinavir plus nucleoside analogues showed good response in late-stage disease. The major problem is resistance, which usually reflects multiple-point mutations on the protease gene. Resistance to indinavir precludes effective future use of this drug, ritonavir, and possibly (codon 82) nelfinavir. The problem with resistance is magnified by monotherapy, noncompliance, failure to use full dosage, or addition of a single drug to a failing regimen.

Dose: 800 mg q8h in fasting stage; always use in combination, usually with a nucleoside analogue; should take >48 oz fluid/day to reduce frequency of nephrolithiasis.

Pharmacology

Bioavailability—Absorption is best with fasting state or with a light meal that does not contain fat

C max = peak >200 nM; 8 hr post dose—80 nM (95% inhibition at 25–100 nM in vitro)

T½ serum—1.5–2 hr

Excretion—Metabolized, especially hepatic glucuronidation and p450 dependent pathways. Urine shows 5–12% unchanged drug and metabolites

Side effects

1. Asymptomatic and clinically inconsequential increase in indirect bilirubin to ≥2.5 mg/dL without increase in transaminase noted in 10–15% of patients.
2. *Nephrolithiasis* ± hematuria in 5–15%. Should take 48 oz fluid daily.

3. Less common: *Hepatitis* with increased transaminase levels, *headache, nausea, vomiting, diarrhea, metallic taste, fatigue, insomnia, blurred vision, dizziness, rash, thrombocytopenia.*

Drug interactions

1. Nucleoside analogues (AZT, ddC, d4T, and 3TC): None known.
2. Other antiretrovirals: Nevirapine—decreases indinavir levels 10–30%—increase indinavir dose to 1000 mg q 8 h; delavirdine—increases indinavir levels 2×—decrease indinavir dose to 400 mg q 8 h; nelfinavir—nelfinavir levels increase 2.5× and indinavir levels increase 50%—dose adjustments are not established; saquinavir—saquinavir levels increase 4–7×—dose adjustment unclear; ritonavir—no data.
3. Ketoconazole: Increases levels of indinavir/70%
4. Rifampin and rifabutin: Decrease levels of indinavir and indinavir increases levels of rifabutin. Concurrent use with rifampin is contraindicated; rifabutin should be reduced to half dose-150 mg/day.
5. Increased levels and potential serious consequences with co-administration with astemizole, cisapride, midazolam, terfenadine, and triazolam; concurrent use is not recommended.
6. ddI given concurrently decreased indinavir absorption; they should be given ≥2 hours apart.

RITONAVIR *Trade name:* Norvir (Abbott)

Form: 100 mg caps

Cost: $1.85/100 mg cap

Clinical trials: Phase I/II trials have shown that ritonavir as a single agent has dose-related antiviral activity with median maximum reductions in viral load of 1.7–1.9 logs at 4–8 weeks and median increases in CD4 counts of 230/mm^3 at 32 weeks (N Engl J Med 1995;333:1534; N Engl J Med 1995;333:1528). A phase-III trial of ritonavir plus nucleoside analogues in 1090 patients with CD4 counts <100/mm^3 showed a 58% decrease in AIDS-defining events or death in ritonavir recipients compared with those continued on nucleoside analogues alone (3rd Conference on Retroviruses and Opportunistic Infections, Washington, DC, Jan 28–Feb 1, 1996, Abstract LB6a). A trial of ritonavir plus

AZT and ddC in treatment-naive patients showed a mean increase in CD4 count of 80–100/mm^3 and a mean reduction in viral burden on 2.9 log. A potent antiviral effect with no detectable virus in >50% of patients has also been achieved with ritonavir plus saquinavir ± nucleosides. The major limitation is resistance ascribed to multiple mutations on the protease gene; there is extensive cross-resistance with indinavir, modest with nelfinavir, minimal with saquinavir, and none with nevirapine or nucleosides.

Dose: 600 mg bid po; dose-escalation regimen—Day 1–2: 300 mg bid; day 3–5: 400 mg bid; day 6–13: 500 mg bid; day ≥14:600 mg bid

Pharmacology

Bioavailability: 60–80%, T½ serum: 3–5 hr

C max: 7–11 mg/mL (2.1 mg/mL = 95% inhibitory concentration); excretion: hepatic metabolism by the cytochrome p450 mechanism. Ritonavir induces its own excretion so that therapeutic levels are achieved with the graduated-dose regimen noted above.

Side effects: Dose related—*GI intolerance* is the major limiting side effect; this often improves with treatment over 1 month and with the graduated-dose regimen noted above. Other side effects include *circumoral* and *peripheral paresthesias* and *increased transaminase levels*. Side effects are sufficiently severe to require discontinuation in 10–30%. Cholesterol levels increase 30–40% and triglyceride levels increase 200–300%. Hepatitis rates increase substantially in patients with chronic HCV or HBV who receive ritonavir plus saquinavir.

Drug interactions: Potent inhibition of p450 enzyme, which contraindicates concurrent use of the following drugs: astemizole, amiodarone, alprazolam (Xanax), bepridil (Vascor), cisapride (Propulsid), clozapine, clorazepate (Tranxene), diazepam (Valium), ergot alkaloids, estazolam (Prosom), encainide, flecainide, flurazepam, meperidine (Demerol), midazolam (Versed), piroxicam (Feldene), pimozide, propoxyphene (Darvon), propafenone, quinidine, rifabutin, terfenadine (Seldane), triazolam (Halcion), and zolpidem (Ambien). Other interactions include increased levels of clarithromycin (CID 1996;23:6); induction of hepatic glucuronyl transferase and CYP1A2 activity results in reduced levels of theophyllin and ethinyl estradiol—alternative methods of birth control should be used. Ritonavir (460–600 mg/day) is commonly combined with saquinavir (400 mg/day) due to a favorable drug interaction.

NELFINAVIR *Trade name:* Viracept (Agouron Pharmaceuticals)

Form: 250 mg caps

Clinical trials: Initial trials show nelfinavir to be very well tolerated: only 4% of 696 patients discontinued treatment due to side effects. Trial 511 compared nelfinavir plus AZT and 3TC vs AZT plus 3TC in 297 treatment-naive patients. This showed triple therapy resulted in no detectable virus in 81% at 24 weeks compared with 18% in recipients of AZT plus 3TC; the average CD4 increase was 155/mm^3. A trial of nelfinavir plus d4T vs d4T alone showed recipients of the former regimen experienced a mean increase in CD4 count of 103/mm^3 and a mean log reduction in viral burden of 1.1 log. Preliminary results of the trial with nelfinavir plus saquinavir looks promising. Resistance to nelfinavir is strongly associated with a codon 30 mutation on the protease gene; this does not confer resistance to other protease inhibitors. There is modest resistance overlap with ritonavir and indinavir by mutations at codons 36, 46, 71, and 82. It is estimated that 60% of clinical HIV isolates from patients who failed treatment with ritonavir or indinavir will be susceptible to nelfinavir.

Dose: 750 mg po q 8 h

Pharmacology: Bioavailability— >70% ± meal, T½ serum: 3.5–5 hr; Excretion: hepatic cytochrome p450, only 1–2% found in urine and up to 90% is found in stool

Side effects: In therapeutic trials, only 28 of 696 (4%) discontinued nelfinavir due to side effects. About 10% of 1500 participants in trials had loose stools, but only 1.6% had diarrhea sufficiently severe to require discontinuation.

Drug interactions: The cytochrome P450 enzyme is inhibited by nelfinavir, primarily CYP3A. *Drugs that must be avoided for concurrent use are* cisapride, astemizole, midazolam, and triazolam. Ketoconazole had no important effect on nelfinavir levels so that azoles and macrolides can presumably be given concurrently in usual doses. Rifampin reduces nelfinavir levels substantially and should not be given concurrently; rifabutin is not problematic for nelfinavir, but rifabutin levels increase 3-fold so that the rifabutin dose should be reduced to half. There are no important drug interactions with nucleoside analogues. Interactions with other nonnucleoside RT inhibitors have not been studied. With regard to protease inhibitors: saquinavir increases nelfinavir levels by about 20%, indinavir by 80%, and ritonavir by 150%. The impact of nelfinavir on these agents is: saquinavir increases 3- to 5-fold, indinavir increases 50%, and ritonavir levels are unchanged. The combination of nelfinavir (750 mg tid) and soft gel cap saquinavir (800 mg tid) is undergoing testing.

NONNUCLEOSIDE REVERSE TRANSCRIPTOR INHIBITOR

NEVIRAPINE *Trade name:* Viramune (Roxane Labs)

Form: 200 mg tabs

Cost: $4.13/200 mg tab

Patient assistance: 800-274-8651

Clinical trials: Nevirapine monotherapy results in a rapid single-point mutation at codon 181 that imparts high-grade resistance. AZT plus nevirapine also results in frequent and rapid evolution of resistance. Optimal results are achieved with combinations that include at least two nucleoside analogues (Ann Intern Med 1996;124:1019).

Dose: 200 mg qd ("lead in" × 2 wks), then 200 mg po bid unless rash precludes standard dose.

Pharmacology: Bioavailability— >90%; average is 93%; T½—25 hr, CSF penetration—45% of serum levels; excretion—biotransformed by hepatic cytochrome p450 enzymes. Nevirapine induces p450 reducing its own half-life so that half-life of 45 hours is reduced to 25 hours.

Side effects: The *major toxicity* is rash seen in about 17%; the usual rash is maculopapular and erythematous with or without pruritus located on the trunk, face, and extremities. Most rashes are seen during the first month, 25% of patients in preclinical trials with rashes required hospitalization, and 7% of all patients required discontinuation of the drug. Indications to discontinue therapy are severe rash, or rash accompanied by fever, blisters, mucous membrane involvement, conjunctivitis, edema, arthralgias, or malaise.

Other side effects include drug-induced hepatitis: discontinue if liver function tests are moderately or severely impaired;

readminister when LFTs return to baseline and discontinue permanently if hepatitis recurs. Additional side effects are fever, nausea, and headache.

Drug interactions: Major concern is induction of cytochrome P450 and metabolism by that mechanism, but there is minimal experience with relevant drugs. Concurrent use with indinavir reduces levels of indinavir 30–40%; the dose of indinavir should be increased to 1000 mg q8h with no dose adjustment of nevirapine. Nevirapine reduces levels of saquinavir so that this combination should be avoided. There is minimal interaction with ritonavir. Concurrent use with rifampin, rifabutin, and oral contraceptives should be done with caution.

DELAVIRDINE *Trade name:* Rescriptor (Pharmacia-Upjohn)

Form: 100 mg tabs

Cost: $0.51/100 mg tab ($6.16/day)

Patient assistance program: 800-711-0807

Clinical trials: Study 0021 showed modest benefit for delavirdine plus AZT versus AZT monotherapy. Study 0071 showed delavirdine plus ddI was therapeutically equivalent to ddI alone. ACTG 261 showed the following regimens were comparable: delavirdine plus AZT, delavirdine plus ddI and AZT plus ddI. A potential advantage of this drug is its interactions to increase levels of saquinavir and indinavir.

Dose: 400 mg po tid dispersed in water.

Pharmacology: Bioavailability—85% (in slurry); T½—5.8 hr; excretion—metabolized by cytochrome p450 enzymes.

Side effects: Rash in 18%; 4% require discontinuation.

Drug interactions: Inhibits cytochrome p450 enzymes. The following are contraindicated for concurrent use—terfenadine, astemizole, alprazolam, midazolam, cisapride, rifabutin, rifampin. Drugs that decrease delavirdine levels: phenytoin, rifabutin, rifampin, carbamazepine, phenobarbitol. Dalavirdine increases levels of the following: dapson, clarithromycin, ergot alkaloids, quinidine, warfarin, indinavir, and saquinavir. Antacids and ddI interfere with absorption and should be separated by ≥ hour.

6—Management of Complications

Table 25. Management of Opportunistic Infections in Patients with HIV Infection

	Preferred	Alternative	Comment
PROTOZOA			
Pneumocystis carinii			
Acute infection	Trimethoprim 15 mg/kg/day + sulfamethoxazole 75 mg/kg/day po or IV × 21 days in 3–4 divided doses	Trimethoprim 15 mg/kg/day po or IV + dapsone 100 mg po/day × 21 days Pentamidine 4 mg/kg/day IV × 21 days Clindamycin 600 mg IV q8h or 300–450 mg po q6h + primaquine[a] 30 mg base po/day × 21 days Atovaquone 750 mg suspension po with meal bid × 21 days Trimetrexate 45 mg/m^2 IV/day plus folinic acid 20 mg/m^2 po or IV q6h ± dapsone 100 mg/day × 21 days	ACTG 108 showed TMP-SMX, trimethoprime-dapsone, and clindamycin-primaquine to be equally effective for mild–moderate PCP (Ann Intern Med 1996; 124:792) Intolerance to TMP-SMX is noted in 25–50%, primarily skin rash ± fever; (Lancet 1991;338:431) Patients with moderately severe or severe disease (pO_2 < 70 mm Hg) should receive corticosteroids (prednisone, 40 mg po bid × 5 days, then 20 mg/day to completion of treatment). Side effects include CNS toxicity, thrush, *H. simplex* infection, tuberculosis, and other OIs (J AIDS 1995;8:345)

Prophylaxis (J AIDS 1993;6:46.)	Trimethoprim (2.5 mg/kg) + sulfamethoxazole po (1 DS/day)	TMP-SMX 1 SS/day or 1 DS 3×/wk Aerosolized pentamidine 300 mg q month via Respirgard II nebulizer ± B_2 agonist (albuterol, 2 puffs) Dapsone 50 mg po bid or 100 mg po qd Dapsone 50 mg/day po plus pyrimethamine 50 mg/wk po plus folinic acid 25 mg/wk po Dapsone 200 mg/wk po plus pyrimethamine 75 mg/wk po + folinic acid 25 mg/wk po Pyrimethamine + sulfadiazine for suppressive treatment of toxoplasmosis is adequate for PCP prophylaxis; pyrimethamine plus clindamycin is not *Other regimens* without established efficacy: Dapsone 50 mg/day po, Pentamidine 4 mg/kg IM or IV q 4 wks, atovaquone 750 mg/day po with meal or Fansidar, 1–2×/wk	*Indications:* history of *Pneumocystis* pneumonia, CD4 count <200/cm mm^3 (or <14%), thrush, or FUO TMP-SMX is superior in efficacy for PCP prophylaxis compared to dapsone and aerosolized pentamidine; TMP-SMX also prevents toxoplasmosis and bacterial infections (NEJM 1995;332:693; NEJM 1992;327:1842) ACTG 021 showed rates of PCP at 12 months were 19% for aerosolized pentamidine vs 4% for TMP-SMX Adverse drug reactions requiring drug discontinuation are noted in 20–40% receiving TMP-SMX, 20–40% receiving dapsone, and 2–5% given aerosolized pentamidine Regimens with dapsone plus pyrimethamine are effective for preventing PCP and toxoplasmosis Patients who have mild or moderate reactions to TMP-SMX may be rechallenged or desensitized

Table 25. *(continued)*

	Preferred	Alternative	Comment
Toxoplasma encephalitis			
Acute infection	Pyrimethamine 100–200 mg loading dose, then 50–100 mg/day po + folinic acid 10 mg/day po + sulfadiazine or trisulfapyrimidine 4–8 g/day po for at least 6 wks	Pyrimethamine + folinic acid (prior doses) + clindamycin 900–1200 mg IV q6h or 300–450 mg po q6h for at least 6 wks Pyrimethamine + folinic acid Azithromycin 900 mg po ×2 1st day, then 1200 mg/day ×6 wks, then 600 mg/day (patients <50 kg receive half dose) (Salvage therapy) Atovaquone 1500 mg po bid or 750 mg po qid and folinic acid for patients who fail or are intolerant of standard treatment (Salvage therapy) Azithromycin IV: 500 mg ×2 on day 1, then 500 mg/d	Patients who respond to primary therapy should receive life-long suppressive therapy Sulfadiazine is available from Eon Labs (718-276-8607) Response: Expect clinical response in 1 wk and MRI or CT scan response at 2 wks Corticosteroids if significant edema/mass effect (Decadron, 4 mg po or IV q6h) Pyrimethamine usually given as a loading dose of 200 mg followed by 50 mg/day plus folinic acid 10 mg/day Controlled trial showed pyrimethamine + sulfa to be superior to pyrimethamine + clindamycin (CID 1996;22: 268)
Suppressive therapy	Pyrimethamine 25–75 mg po qd + folinic acid 10 mg qd + sulfadiazine 0.5–1.0 g po q6h	Pyrimethamine 25–75 mg/day po + folinic acid 10–25 mg qd to qid + clindamycin 300–450 mg po q6–8h	Pyrimethamine—sulfadiazine is effective prophylaxis for PCP, pyrimethamine-clindamycin is not.

		Regimen without established merit Pyrimethamine 25–75 mg/day po + folinic acid 10–25 mg qd or qid + either Atovaquone 750 mg/day bid po, Dapsone 100 mg/day po, or Azithromycin 500 mg/day po *Other agents* without established efficacy include atovaquone, trimethoprim-sulfa, azithromycin, clarithromycin, and trimetrexate	
Prophylaxis (See comment)	Trimethoprim-sulfamethoxazole 1 DS po qd	TMP-SMX 1 SS/day po or 1 DS 3×/wk Dapsone 50 mg/day po + pyrimethamine 50 mg/wk po + folinic acid 25 mg/wk po Dapsone 200 mg/wk po + pyrimethamine 75 mg/wk po + folinic acid 25 mg/wk po *Other regimens without established efficacy:* pyrimethamine-clindamycin, atovaquone, azithromycin or pyrimethamine-sulfadoxine (Fansidar)	*Indications:* patients with positive toxoplasmosis IgG serology plus CD4 count $<100/mm^3$ Efficacy for prophylaxis is established for TMP-SMX and Dapsone + pyrimethamine Pyrimethamine 25 mg 3×/wk is ineffective; efficacy of 25 mg po qd is not established

Table 25. ***(continued)***

	Preferred	Alternative	Comment
Cryptosporidia	Paromomycin 500 mg po qid with food × 14–28 days, then 500 mg po bid Symptomatic treatment with nutritional supplements and antidiarrheal agents: Lomotil, loperamide, paregoric, bismuth subsalicylate (Pepto Bismol) Nitrazoxanide 1000 mg/d	Octreotide (Sandostatin) 50–500 μg tid SC or IV at 1 mcg/hr Azithromycin 1200 mg ×2 po 1st day, then 1200 mg/day × 27 days, then 600 mg/day Atovaquone 750 mg po suspension with meal bid	Efficacy of atovaquone and azithromycin not established; other possibly effective agent: Hyperimmune colostrum Non-steroidal anti-inflammatory agents sometimes useful Nutritional supplements often required for severe cases: Vivonex TEN or parenteral hyperalimentation Paromomycin is only modestly effective (Am J Med 1996; 100:370)
Isospora			
Acute infection	Trimethoprim + sulfamethoxazole po bid (2 DS po bid or 1 DS tid) ×2–4 wks	Pyrimethamine 50–75 mg po/day + folinic acid 5–10 mg/day ×1 mo	Duration of high-dose therapy is not well defined
Suppressive treatment	Trimethoprim + Sulfamethoxazole 1–2 DS/day po	Pyrimethamine 25 mg + sulfadoxine 500 mg po q wk (1 Fansidar/wk) Pyrimethamine 25 mg + folinic acid 5 mg/day	Duration is not well defined

Microsporidiosis	Albendazole 400 mg po bid ≥4 wks Symptomatic treatment with nutritional supplements and anti-diarrheal agents (Lomotil, loperamide, paregoric, etc.)	Metronidazole 500 mg po tid Atovaquone 750 mg po with meals bid	Efficacy of albendazole suggested in uncontrolled trial (JID: 1994;169:178) Higher doses (800 mg bid) of albendazole may be required Anecdotal success with itraconazole capsules, fluconazole, atovaquone, and metronidazole (Inf Dis Clin North Am 1994;8:483)
FUNGI			
Aspergillosis			
Pulmonary infection	Amphotericin B: 1.0—1.4 mg/kg/day ± flucytosine 100 mg/kg/day	Itraconazole capsules 200 mg po bid Amphotericin B Lipid Complex (Abelcet) 5 mg/kg/day	Total dose of Amphotericin B: 30–40 mg/kg Long-term maintenance is usually not necessary Predisposing factors: Corticosteroids (decrease or stop if possible); neutropenia: G-CSF and avoid 5-FC; marijuana Amphotericin B Lipid Complex. Advantage is reduced nephrotoxicity, but cost is high—$430/treatment compared to $21/50 mg Amphotericin B

Table 25. *(continued)*

	Preferred	Alternative	Comment
Candida			
Thrush			
Initial infection	Nystatin 500,000 units gargled 5×/day Clotrimazole oral 10 mg troches 5×/day; Fluconazole 100 mg/day po Itraconazole oral solution 100 mg/day	Amphotericin B 0.3–0.5 mg/kg IV/day Itraconazole capsules 200 mg/day Amphotericin B oral suspension 1 mL qid swish & swollow	Treat until symptoms resolve (usually 7–14 days) Fluconazole 100 mg/d and itraconazole capsules 200 mg/day or oral solution 100 mg/day are comparable to ketoconazole 400 mg/d in efficacy and show reduced side effects (Rev Infect Dis 1990;12;S364) Amphotericin B usually reserved for patients who fail with oral regimens; most common with chronic azole administration and azole-resistant *Candida sp.*
Maintenance (optional or prn: see comment)	Nystatin, clotrimazole Fluconazole 100 mg/day po or 200 mg 3×/wk	Itraconazole capsules 100 mg/day or Itraconazole oral solution 100 mg qod Ketoconazole 200 mg/day po	Salutary advantage of fluconazole for maintenance treatment is prevention of deep fungal infection: cryptococcosis and *Candida* esophagitis with CD4 count <100/mm^3 (N Engl J Med 332:700, 1995) Fluconazole is superior to clotrimazole in preventing relapses of thrush

			Most patients will have relapse within 3 mo past therapy if treatment is discontinued. Options are to treat each episode of maintenance. Concerns with continuous treatment with fluconazole are azole resistance by *Candida sp.*, drug interactions and cost; maintenance treatment recommended if recurrences are frequent or severe. (CID 21 Suppl 1:518, 1995; JID 1996;173:219)
Prophylaxis	Not recommended		Efficacy of fluconazole (100 mg bid po) is established for AIDS patients with CD4 counts <100/mm^3; this is not generally advocated because the study showd no survival benefit, treatment of cryptococcosis is generally effective, the cost is high and there is concern for azole-resistant *Candida* infections (N Engl J Med 1995;332:700)
Vaginitis	Intravaginal miconazole 200 mg suppository or 2% cream ×7 days; Clotrimazole 1% cream or 100 mg tab qd ×7 days or 100 mg ×2/d ×3 days or 500 mg × 1	Ketoconazole[b] 200 mg/day po or bid × 5–7 days or 200 mg po bid × 3 days Intraconazole capsules 200 mg bid × 1 day or 200 mg/d × 3 days	May require continuous treatment to prevent relapse: ketoconazole 100 mg/day po or fluconazole 50–100 mg/day or 200 mg/week po

Table 25. ***(continued)***

	Preferred	Alternative	Comment
	Fluconazole 150 mg po ×1		Clotrimazole and miconazole (both cream and 100 mg tabs) are available over-the-counter
Esophagitis Initial infection	Fluconazole 200 mg/day po; up to 400 mg/day × 2–3 wks Itraconazole oral solution 100–200 mg/day	Ketoconazole[b] 200–400 mg po bid × 2–3 wks Itraconazole capsules 100–200 mg tab po bid Amphotericin B 0.3—0.5 mg/kg/day ± flucytosine 100 mg/kg/day × 5–7 days	Fluconazole is clinically superior to ketoconazole as initial treatment Relapse rate is 84% within one year without prophylaxis
Maintenance	Fluconazole 100–200 mg/day po	Ketoconazole[b] 200 mg/day po Itraconazole capsules 200 mg/day or Itraconazole oral solution 100 mg/day Nystatin (above dose) or clotrimazole (above doses)	Recommended only if subsequent episodes are frequent or severe
Cryptococcal meningitis Initial treatment	Amphotericin B 0.5–1.0 mg/kg/day IV to complete 700 mg–1 gm of Amphotericin B or until 15 mg/kg plus sterile CSF Amphotericin B 0.7 mg/kg/day IV × 10–14 days, ± flucytosine 100 mg/kg/day	Fluconazole 400 mg/day po × 6–10 wks Itraconazole capsules 200 mg tid × 3 days, then 200 mg po bid (see comment) Fluconazole 400 mg/d po plus flucytosine 100 mg/kg/day po	LP with fluid withdrawal (25–30 ml) with symptomatic increased intracranial pressure qd or prn Amphotericin B is preferred for initial treatment, but total dose prior to fluconazole maintenance is arbitrary

	po, then fluconazole 400 mg/day × 8–10 wks		Fluconazole is acceptable as initial treatment only for patients with normal mental status. Other favorable prognostic findings are crypt antigen <1:32 and CSR WBC >20/mm^3 Cryptococcal antigen is nearly always detected in CSF and is somewhat useful in monitoring response; sensitivity of *serum* antigen is 95%; but it is less useful in monitoring response Efficacy of Itraconazole capsules not established and CNS penetration is poor. Dose of the oral solution is half the capsule dose Fluconazole may be used in dose up to 800 mg/day for salvage therapy Addition of 5FU to Amphotericin appears to be of little value and associated with high rates of toxicity
Maintenance therapy	Fluconazole 200 mg/day po up to 400 mg/day	Amphotericin B 0.6–1 mg/kg 1–3×/wk Itraconazole capsules 400 mg/day or Itraconazole oral solution 200 mg/d	Lifelong maintenance treatment required for all patients Itraconazole capsules, in doses of 200 mg/d, is inadequate; trial with 400 mg/d is ongoing

Table 25. ***(continued)***

	Preferred	Alternative	Comment
Prophylaxis (see comment)	Fluconazole 200 mg/day po	Itraconazole capsules 200 mg/day or Itraconazole oral solution 100 mg/day	*Indications:* USPHS/IDSA Guidelines recommend only for selected patients plus CD4 count <50/mm³. Concerns are: most deep fungal infections are easily treated. Cryptococcosis is infrequent (8–10%), potential for azole-resistant *Candida*, drug interactions and cost
Cryptococcosis without meningitis (pulmonary or disseminated) or antigenemia	Regimens for cryptococcal meningitis Fluconazole 200 mg po bid × 6–10 wks	Itraconazole capsules 200 mg bid or Itraconazole oral solution 100 mg/day × 6–10 wks	All patients with cryptococcosis should have LP to exclude meningitis Antigenemia: chest x ray, LP, urine and blood culture. If no focus and antigenemia persists: treat with fluconazole
Maintenance	Fluconazole 200 mg/day po	Itraconazole capsules 200 mg/day or Itraconazole oral solution 100 mg/d Amphotericin B 0.6–1 mg/kg IV weekly or 2×/wk	Need for maintenance treatment is not established

Histoplasmosis			
Disseminated			
Initial treatment	Amphotericin B 0.5–1.0 mg/kg/day IV × ≥7–14 Itraconazole capsules 200 mg tid × 3 days; then 200 mg capsules bid or half dose in Itraconazole oral solution	Fluconazole 400 mg po qd	Itraconazole capsules or oral solution may be used for initial treatment of mild to moderate histoplasmosis without CNS involvement or it may be used for maintenance after induction with Amphotericin B (Am J Med 1995;98:336)
Maintenance	Itraconazole capsules 200 mg bid or Itraconazole oral solution 100 mg bid	Amphotericin B 1.0 mg/kg/wk Fluconazole 200–400 mg/day po	Efficacy of itraconazole is established (Ann Intern Med 1993;118:610). Efficacy of fluconazole is not established
Prophylaxis	Itraconazole capsules 200 mg/d or Itraconazole oral solution 100 mg/d	Fluconazole 200 mg/day po	*Indication:* Consider in endemic area with CD4 <50/mm^3
Coccidioidomycosis			
Initial treatment	Amphotericin B 0.5–1.0 mg/kg iV/day × ≥8 wks (2–2.5 g total dose)	Fluconazole 400 mg po qd Itraconazole capsules 200 mg bid or Itraconazole oral solution 100 mg bid	Intrathecal Amphotericin B usually added for coccidioidomycosis meningitis
Maintenance	Fluconazole 200 mg/day	Amphotericin B 1 mg/kg/wk Ketoconazole 400–800 mg/day po Itraconazole capsules 200 mg bid or oral solution 100 mg bid	
Prophylaxis	Fluconazole 200 mg/day po	Itraconazole capsules 200 mg qd or oral solution 100 mg/day	*Indications:* Consider in endemic area with CD4 <50/mm^3
Penicillium marneffei	Amphotericin B 0.7–1.0 mg/kg/d Itraconazole-400 mg po/d; maintenance-200–400 mg/d	Fluconazole	Fever ± pneumonitis, adenopathy, skin lesions Endemic regions: Thailand, Africa, Hong Kong, and Indonesia

Table 25. *(continued)*

	Preferred	Alternative	Comment

MYCOBACTERIA
M. tuberculosis
Treatment
(Revised ATS guide-lines, AM J Crit Care Med 149: 1359, 1994)

Preferred

Directly observed treatment (DOT) 2–3×/wk preferred
Doses

	Daily	DOT 2×/wk	DOT 3×/wk
INH	5 mg/kg (300 mg)*	15 mg/kg (900 mg)*	15 mg/kg (900 mg)*
Rif	10 mg/kg (600 mg)*	10 mg/kg (600 mg)*	10 mg/kg (600 mg)*
PZA	15–30 mg/kg (2 g)*	50–70 mg/kg (4 g)*	50–70 mg/kg (3 g)*
EMB	15–25 mg/kg (2.5 g)	50 mg/kg (2.5 g)*	25–30 mg/kg (2.5 g)*
Strep	15 mg/kg (1 g)*	25–30 mg/kg (1.5 g)*	25–30 mg/kg (1 g)*

* Maximum dose

Duration: 6 months

Option 1: INH, Rif, PZA + SM or EMB daily × 8 wks, then INH + Rif daily or DOT × 16 weeks if isolate sensitive to INH and Rif

Option 2: INH, Rif, PZA + SM or EMB daily × 2 wks, then DOT with same 4 drugs × 6 wks, then INH + Rif × 16 weeks if isolate sensitive to INH and Rif

Option 3: INH, Rif, PZA + SM or EMB by DOT 3×/wk × 6 mo

Monitoring: Smear or culture positive or symptomatic at 2 months—consult expert

Alternative

Second line drugs: Ethionamide 1 g/day po, capreomycin 15–30 mg/kg IM or IV (maximum dose—1 g), cycloserine 250–500 mg po bid, kanamycin 15–30 mg/kg/day IM or IV/day (maximum dose–1 g), PAS 150 mg/kg/day po (maximum dose—12 g/day)

Experimental drugs: Ofloxacin 600 mg/day po or Ciprofloxacin 1–1.5 g/day po, clofazimine 100–200 mg/day po, amikacin 15 mg/kg/day IM or IV (maximum dose—1 g)

Comment

Observed treatment preferred for all patients

Intermittent treatment: 2×/wk appears to be as effective as 3×/wk

INH: Should supplement with pyridoxine (50 mg/day) in AIDS patients

Resistance to INH: Rif + EMB ± PZA × 12 mo

Multiply resistant strains: (N Engl J Med 329:784, 1993)

Resistant to	Regimen suggested
INH, strep, PZA	Rif, PZA, EMB, Amik*
INH, EMB ± strep	Rif, PZA, Cipro or Oflox, Amik*
INH + Rif	PZA, EMB, Cipro or Oflox, Amik*
INH, Rif, EMB + Strep	PZA, Cipro or Oflox, Amik* + 2†
INH, Rif, PZA ± Strep	EMB, Cipro or Oflox, Amik* + 2†
INH, Rif, PLZA, EMB ± strep	Cipro or Oflox, Amik* + 3†

* Aminoglycoside (amikacin, strep, kanamycin, capreomycin) based on in vitro sensitivity, given daily, 2×/wk or 3×/wk IM or IV × 4–6 mo

† Ethionamide, cycloserine, PAS, clofazimine(?) or Augmentin(?)

			Improved outcome in HIV-infected patients with MDR-TB who are treated with ≥2 drugs active in vitro; median survival was 6.8 mo (Am J Respir Crit Care Med 153: 317,1996) Aminoglycoside: streptomycin usually preferred and may be given IV; capreomycin, kanamycin, or amikacin may be preferred based on in vitro sensitivity tests Suspected resistance: Give 3 drugs never seen pending in vitro sensitivity tests; never add a single drug
Prophylaxis INH-sensitive strain	INH 300 mg/day po + pyridoxine 50 mg/day po × 12 mo	Rifampin 600 mg po qd × 12 mo	*Indications:* PPD > 5 mm, high-risk exposure or prior positive PPD without treatment Pyridoxine (50 mg/day) advocated for all HIV-infected patients given INH
INH-resistant strain or INH intolerance	Rifampin 600 mg/day po × 12 mo		
Multiply resistant strain	Two of the 3 following agents: Fluroquinolones, pyrazinamide, ethambutol	Rifabutin 600 mg po qd × 12 mo	Base decision on sensitivity tests and consultation with public health officials
M. avium-complex Treatment	Clarithromycin 500 mg po bid plus ethambutol 15 mg/kg/day po ± rifabutin 300 mg/day po or ciprofloxacin 500–750 mg bid po	Azithromycin 500 mg/day po in place of clarithromycin plus one or more of the drugs listed in the preferred treatment column Combination treatment with amikacin 10–15 mg/kg/day IV or clofazimine 100 mg/day IV	Clarithromycin is only drug that shows correlation between in vitro activity and clinical plus microbiological response Clarithromycin dose >500 mg bid is associated with increased mortality Clofazimine is no longer

Table 25. ***(continued)***

	Preferred	Alternative	Comment
			recommended (N Engl J Med 1996;335:377) Rifabutin dose is 300–600 mg/day, but should not exceed 300 mg/day if given with clarithromycin or fluconazole ASA or NSAID often effective for symptom relief
Prophylaxis	Clarithromycin 500 mg po bid Azithromycin 1200 mg po q wk	Rifabutin 300 mg/day po Rifabutin 300 mg/day po + clarithromycin 500 mg po bid or azithromycin 1200 mg po/wk	*Indications:* USPHS/IDSA Guidelines recommend prophylaxis with CD4 <100/mm^3; rule out MAC bacteremia and active TB Clarithromycin and azithromycin have established efficacy for MAC prophylaxis, and both have proven superior to rifabutin in comparative trials Prophylaxis failures with rifabutin usually involve rifabutin-resistant strains; failures with clarithromycin may involve clarithromycin-resistant strains
M. kansasii	INH 300 mg po/day + rifampin 600 mg po/day + ethambutol 15–25 mg/kg po/day × 18 mo and for at least 15 months post sputum conversion ± streptomycin 1 g IM 2×/wk × 3 mo	Also consider ciprofloxacin 750 mg po bid and clarithromycin 500 mg—1 g po bid	Experience is limited

VIRUSES			
Herpes simplex			
Initial treatment			
Mild	Acyclovir 400 mg po 3×/day at least 10 days or until lesions crusted		Failure to respond: double oral dose or give IV
Severe or refractory	Acyclovir 15 mg/kg IV/day or 800 mg po 5×/day at least 7 days	Foscarnet 40 mg/kg IV q8h or 60 mg/kg q12h × 3 wks Topical trifluridine 1% ophthalmic solution q8h	If fails to respond to acyclovir give 30 mg/kg/day IV and test sensitivity of isolate to acyclovir. Acyclovir-resistant HSV: IV foscarnet, topical trifluridine, or high-dose IV acyclovir (12–15 mg/kg IV q8h or by continuous infusion). (J AIDS 7:254, 1994). Relapses after treatment of acyclovir-resistant strains often involve acyclovir-sensitive strains Topical trifluridine solution (Viroptic 1%) is applied after H_2O_2 cleansing and gentle gauze debridement; cover with non-absorbable gauze with bacitracin and polymyxin ointment
Maintenance	Acyclovir 400 mg po bid or 400 mg 3–5×/day	Foscarnet 40 mg/kg IV/day	Indication is ≥6 outbreaks/year or chronic HSV infection Alternative is to treat each episode Patients receiving ganciclovir or foscarnet treatment do not need acyclovir
Visceral HSV infection	Acyclovir 30 mg/kg IV/day at least 10 days	Foscarnet 40 mg/kg IV q8h × ≥10 days	

Table 25. *(continued)*

	Preferred	Alternative	Comment
Herpes zoster			
Dermatomal	Acyclovir 30 mg/kg IV/day or 800 mg po 5×/day at least 7 days (until lesions crust)	Foscarnet 40 mg/kg IV q8h or 60 mg/kg IV q12h	Use of steroids is controversial (N Engl J Med 330:896, 1994); post-herpetic neuralgia is less common in young patients; no maintenance therapy recommended Foscarnet preferred for acyclovir-resistant cases Post herpetic neuralgia: nortriptyline or amitriptyline 10–25 mg increasing over 1–2 weeks up to 75–100 mg/day
Disseminated, ophthalmic nerve involvement or visceral	Acyclovir 30–36 mg/kg IV/day at least 7 days	Foscarnet 40 mg/kg IV q8h or 60 mg/kg q12h	Role of maintenance therapy unclear
Acyclovir-resistant strains	Foscarnet 40 mg/kg IV q8h or 60 mg IV q12h		
Maintenance (see comment)	Acyclovir 800 mg po 5×/day		Indication: frequent recurrences

Cytomegalovirus (Retinitis or other end-organ disease) Initial treatment (JAMA 1995;273:1457)	Foscarnet 60 mg/kg IV q8h or 90 mg/kg IV q12h × 14–21 days Ganciclovir 5 mg/kg IV bid × 14–21 days Intraocular Mark II ganciclovir release device (1–2 μg/hr) + oral ganciclovir 1 g po with meal tid Cidofovir 5 mg/kg IV q week ×2, then 5 mg/kg q 2 wks plus probenecid 2 g po 3 hr before each dose, then 1 g po at 2 + hr	Alternating or combinations of foscarnet and ganciclovir Intraocular injection of foscarnet (2400 μg in 0.1 mL) (N Engl J Med 1994;330: 868) or ganciclovir (2 mg) 2–3×/wk for induction and then weekly for maintenance	Ganciclovir and foscarnet appear comparably effective vs CMV with median times to progression of 50–70 days. Possible advantage of foscarnet was prolonged survival ascribed to concurrent use with AZT or activity of foscarnet plus AZT versus HIV (N Engl J Med 326:213, 1992; Am J Med 94:175, 1993) Foscarnet requires infusion pump, long infusion time, saline hydration; cost is high Mark II device shows substantial delay in time to progression (226 days) but 50% risk of CMV retinitis in contralateral eye or visceral CMV disease (Arch Ophthalmol 112:1531, 1994). Many favor concurrent use of oral ganciclovir to protect other eye and prevent systemic CMV disease Cidofovir: Average time to relapse is 115 days (Ann Intern Med 1997;126:257)

Table 25. *(continued)*

	Preferred	Alternative	Comment
Progression (on maintenance therapy)	Increase dose of same agent (ganciclovir 10 mg/kg/d *or* switch to alternative agent (induction doses) Combination treatment with ganciclovir plus foscarnet in maintenance doses (JID 168:444; 1993; Am J Oph 117:776, 1994)		Time to relapse varies with criteria, use of retinal photographs and treatment; with ``standard treatment'' using IV ganciclovir or foscarnet the mean is 50–70 days; subsequent relapses occur earlier
Maintenance	Foscarnet 90–120 mg/kg IV/day Ganciclovir 5–6 mg/kg IV/day 5–7 days/wk Intraocular ganciclovir device q 6 mo. ± oral ganciclovir 1 g po tid Cidofovir 5 mg/kg IV q 2 wks		Indications: maintenance therapy required lifelong for retinitis; indications with other end-organ disease is less well defined Foscarnet maintenance dose is arbitrary; one study showed 120 mg/kg/d was superior to 90 mg/kg/d in survival and time to progression (JID 167:1184, 1993) Comparative trial showed relapses with oral ganciclovir occurred an average of 10–15 days earlier compared to IV ganciclovir

Prophylaxis	Oral ganciclovir 1 g po with meal tid		*Indications:* Efficacy shown in one study of patients with CD4 counts <50 but: cost is high ($15,000/yr), and there is concern about promoting resistance. USPHS/IDSA Guidelines do not recommend prophylactic oral ganciclovir
BACTERIA			
S. pneumoniae			
Treatment	Penicillin, Cefotaxime or Ceftriaxone Penicillin resistant: Vancomycin Cefotaxime, Ceftriaxone, Levofloxacin	Erythromycin Cephalosporins (other) Doxycycline Azithromycin Clarithromycin	Rates of pen-resistance average >25% in U.S.; rates of resistance to macrolides, cephalosporins and TMP-SMX are 10–25% (N Engl J Med 333:48, 1995) Vancomycin is always active; fluoroquinolones are usually active
Prevention	Pneumococcal vaccine 0.5 mL SC		
H. influenzae	Cephalosporins, (2nd & 3rd generation)	Trimethoprim-sulfamethoxazole Fluoroquinolones	Traditional therapy usually adequate
Nocardia asteroids	Sulfadiazine or trisulfapyridine 4–8 g po or IV/day to maintain sulfa level at 15–20 mcg/mL	Trimethoprim-sulfa 4–6 DS/day Minocycline 100 mg po bid	Other suggested regimens: imipenem + amikacin; Sulfonamide + amikacin or minocycline

Table 25. *(continued)*

	Preferred	Alternative	Comment
Pseudomonas aeruginosa	Aminoglycoside + antipseudomonal penicillin (ticarcillin, piperacillin, or mezlocillin)	Aminoglycoside + antipseudomonal cephalosporin (ceftazidime or cefoperazone) or imipenem	Antibiotic selection requires in vitro sensitivity data
Rhodococcus equi	Vancomycin 2 g IV/day ± rifampin 600 mg po qd, ciprofloxacin 750 mg po bid, or imipenem 0.5 g IV qid × 2–4 wks	Erythromycin 2–4 g IV/day	Ciprofloxacin 750 mg po bid may be used for long-term maintenance, but resistance likely to develop
Bartonella henselae/quintana (bacillary angiomatosis)	Erythromycin 250–500 mg po qid × ≥8 wks	Doxycycline 100 mg po bid	
Salmonella			
Acute	Ciprofloxacin 500 po bid × 2–4 wks	Ampicillin 8–12 g IV/day × 1–4 wks; then amoxicillin 500 mg po tid to complete 2–4 wk course Trimethoprim 5–10 mg/kg/day + sulfamethoxazole IV or po × 2–4 wks Cephalosporins, 3rd generation	Relapse common AZT is active vs. most strains of *Salmonella* and may be effective prophylaxis Drug selection requires in vitro susceptibility data especially for ampicillin
Maintenance	Ciprofloxacin 500 mg po bid × several months	Trimethoprim-sulfamethoxazole 5 mg/kg/day trimethoprim (1 DS po bid)	USPHS/IDSA Guidelines recommend ciprofloxacin for ''several months''

Staph. aureus	Antistaphylococcal penicillin IV (nafcillin, oxacillin) ± gentamicin 1 mg/kg IV q8h or rifampin 300 mg po bid	Cephalosporin: first generation ± gentamicin or rifampin	MRSA strains must be treated with vancomycin
	Oral agents: Cephalexin 500 mg po qid, dicloxacillin 500 mg po qid, ciprofloxacin 750 mg po bid		
	Tricuspid valve endocarditis: Ciprofloxacin 750 mg po bid + rifampin 300 mg po bid *or* oxacillin 3 gm IV q6h + gentamicin 1 mg/kg IV q8h	Vancomycin 1 g IV bid ± gentamicin 1 mg/kg IV q8h or rifampin 300 mg po bid	In vitro sensitivity tests required
Treponema pallidum (MMWR 42 RR-14;38–39, 1993)	Primary secondary, or latent syphilis: benzathine penicillin G, 2.4 mil units IM weekly × 3 (see comment)	No alternative considered adequate for HIV-infected patients; with a history of penicillin allergy-skin test if reagent (major and minor) available; if positive skin test or positive history and no skin test: desensitize	Follow-up clinically and serologically at 1, 2, 3, 6, 9, and 12 months
	Neurosyphilis: aqueous penicillin G, 12–24 mil units/day IV × 10–14 days (2–4 mil units q4h)		LP should be encouraged in all HIV-infected patients with syphilis. Treatment for presumed neurosyphilis should be encouraged if CSF is not evaluated

[a] Patients with severe forms of G6PD deficiency are at risk for hemolytic anemia when given oxidant drugs such as dapsone, sulfonamides, and primaquine. Some advocate screening all potential recipients, some restrict screening to persons at greatest risk (African-American men and men of Mediterranean descent, from India, or from the Far East; some simply observe for evidence of hemolysis that usally occurs in first several days of treatment and often resolves with continued administration. Patients with the Mediterranean variant are at risk for severe hemolysis.

[b] Ketoconazole and, to a lesser extent, itraconazole capsules require gastric acid for absorption; absorption with hypochlorhydria may be enhanced by administration with 0.2 N HCl or 240 mL of the following soft drinks which have a pH <3.0: Coca Cola, Pepsi, diet Coke, ginger ale, diet Minute-Maid orange juice (AAC 39:1671, 1995). Itraconazole oral solution is less reliant on gastric acidity for absorption and can be taken with or without food.

Table 26. Treatment of Miscellaneous and Noninfectious Disease Complications of HIV Infection Classified by Organ System

Condition	Treatment	Comment
Cardiac		
Cardiomyopathy	Digitalis, diuretic, and cautious use ACE-inhibitor plus isosorbide Discontinue nucleoside (AZT, ddI or ddC) × 4 wks. (Some patients respond to AZT treatment)	Echo is best screening test. If patient does not respond to nucleoside withdrawal and has severe dysfunction (NYHA class III): prednisone 1 mg/kg/d × 30 days, then taper over one month. Efficacy is not established. Endomyocardial biopsy is another option and may detect microbial agent (CMV, *M. avium*, cryptococcus): treat accordingly.
Pulmonary		
Lymphoid interstitial pneumonitis	AZT Prednisone	Relatively rare in adult patients. Indications and optimal dose of corticosteroid treatment not established; most initiate this treatment after initial observation shows progression; maintenance prednisone sometimes required.
Renal		
Nephropathy (HIV-associated nephropathy (HIVAN))	AZT 600 mg/day Hemodialysis (utility of dialysis in preventing rapid progression of HIVAN is not established) Prednisone 60 mg/day × 2–11 wks, then taper over 2–26 wks (Am J Med 1996;101:41)	Must distinguish from: 1) heroin-associated nephropathy which has a far better prognosis and 2) acute tubular necrosis
Neurologic		
Peripheral neuropathy (painful peripheral)	Nortriptyline 10 mg hs; increase dose by 10 mg q5 days to maximum of 50 mg hs or 10–20 mg po tid Ibuprofen 600–800 mg tid Topical: Capsaicin-containing ointments (Zostrix, etc.) for topical application; Lidocaine 10–30% ointment for topical use.	Other tricyclics are also effective: amitriptyline, desipramine or imipramine. Capsaicin is usually not well tolerated

	Alternatives: Phenytoin 200–400 mg/d, carbamazepine 200–400 mg po bid	
Myopathy	Discontinue AZT × 3 weeks. Nonsteroidal anti-inflammatory agents. See section on "pain control" (pg 111). Prednisone, 40–60 mg/day (severe case, biopsy-proven inflammation)	Indication for treatment is proximal muscle weakness plus elevated creatinekinase. Often unclear if due to HIV or AZT, so use "drug holiday" and monitor clinical and CPK response.
HIV-associated dementia (HAD)	AZT 1000–1200 po/day d4T 40 mg po bid (efficacy not established) Alternative: Nimodipine (calcium channel blocker) 30 mg po q4h (experimental for this indication)	Benefit of AZT at higher dose for mild or moderately severe HAD is established; monitor therapy with neurocognitive tests CNS penetration of d4T is less than AZT, but superior to ddI, ddC or 3TC Penetration across blood-brain barrier is good for AZT, nevirapine, d4T, and hydroxyurea; it is modest for indinavir and nelfinavir
Hematologic		
Idiopathic thrombocytopenia (ITP)		
Asymptomatic	AZT, 600–1200 mg/day Discontinue any drug-related cause	Note: Standard treatments (prednisone, IVIG, splenectomy, etc) show response rates of 40–90%; main problem is lack of a durable response (See CID 1995;21:415). Response to AZT may be dose-related; usually responds within 2–4 wks. Utility of other nucleoside analogs is unknown.
Severe hemorrhage	Packed red cells, platelet transfusions *plus* prednisone 60–100 mg/d or IVIG 1 g/kg days 1, 2, 14 and then q2–3 weeks	
Persistent symptomatic ITP	AZT, 600–1200 mg/day Discontinue drugs potentially responsible and avoid non-steroidal anti-inflammatory agents Prednisone 30–60 mg/day with rapid taper to 5–10 mg/day IVIG 1 g/kg days 1, 2, 14 then q2–3 wks or Win Rho 5 μg/kg IV over 3–5 min; repeat day 3–4 prn Splenectomy	Usual dose is 500–600 mg/day; doses of 1000–1200 mg/day are reserved for non-responders. Response is noted in 2–4 wks. Prednisone may be complicated by OIs, esp. thrush and herpes, and decreased CD4 count; only 10–20% have persistent response. IVIG is very highly effective in raising platelet count within 4 days, *but* is very expensive and median duration of response is only 3 weeks.

Table 26. ***(continued)***

Condition	Treatment	Comment
	Alternatives: Spleen irradiation, danazol, vincristine, interferon	Experience with splenectomy is variable: durability of response is variable and some claim risk of HIV progression is increased (Lancet 1987;2:342) and others claim good long term results (Arch Surg 1989;124:625).
Anemia	Transfusions and/or erythropoietin (r HuEPO) 100–200 U/kg 3×/wk SC; increase dose 50–100 U/kg if response is inadequate at 4–8 wks and again at 4–8 wk intervals; maximum dose is 300 U/kg; titrate maintenance dose—usually 24,000–48,000 U/wk	Discontinue AZT for hemoglobulin <7.5 g/dl. EPO recommended only if baseline EPO level is <500 U/ml and hematocrit <30%. Usual maintenance dose of EPO is 100–200 U/kg 3×/wk; efficacy is established (Oncol Clin N Amer 1991;5:267).
Neutropenia	Neupogen (G-CSF) 5–10 μg/kg SC qd × 2–4 wks or GM-CSF, 250 μg/m² IV over 2 hr qd × 2–4 wks Discontinue AZT, ganciclovir or other marrow-suppressing agent; if critical give concurrent G-CSF	Usual cause is AZT, ganciclovir, or HIV *per se*. Low dose (1 μg/kg/day) of G-CSF is often adequate; monitor with CBC and dif 2×/wk and titrate up to 10 μg/kg; reduce dose 50% q week for maintenance to keep ANC >500–1500/ml. Efficacy of G-CSF or GM-CSF is established for elevating neutrophil count (NEJM 1987;317:593). USPHS/ISDSA Guidelines do not recommend cytokines for neutropenia except in selected patients. Dose of GM-CSF is same as for G-CSF
Thrombotic thrombocytopenic purpura	Prednisone 60–100 mg/day plus plasmapheresis	

Tumors		
Kaposi sarcoma		
Local Treatment	Topical liquid nitrogen	Restrict to few lesions that are small
	Intralesional vinblastine (0.01–0.02 mg/lesion) every 2 wks × ≤3	Restrict to few lesions that may be larger (>1 cm)
	Radiation (low dose, e.g., 400 rads q wk × 6 wks)	Skin—well tolerated; Oral lesion—mucositis common
	Laser	Laser, radiation, or vinblastine injection preferred for oral lesions
Systemic treatment	Chemotherapy: Adriamycin, bleomycin, and either vincristine or vinblastine (ABV); Etoposide (VP-16) monotherapy.	Systemic therapy is preferred for patients with widespread skin involvement (>25 lesions), extensive cutaneous KS that is non-responsive to local treatment, extensive edema and/or symptomatic visceral organ involvement (especially lung KS).
	Liposomal daunorubicin (Daunoxome) 40–60 mg/m^2 IV q2 wks	Alternative to ABV which shows comparable efficacy and reduced toxicity
	Alpha interferon (18–36 million IU/day) IM or SC × 10–12 wks, then 18 million units/day—36 million units 3×/wk.	Response rates better for patients with CD4 count $>200/mm^3$, neutropenia common with AZT: Use G-CSF or substitute other agent.
	Experimental: Paclitaxel (Taxol) for visceral KS, esp. pulmonary involvement; intralesional B-human chorionic gonadotropin 2000 U per lesion; retinoic acid isomers	
Lymphoma	Regimens containing methotrexate, bleomycin, doxorubicin, cyclophosphamide, adriamycin, vincristine, and corticosteroids ± cranial radiation; standard regimens are CHOP and mBACOD + G-CSF.	Low dose chemotherapy is as effective as standard dose (ACTG 142).
	CNS lymphoma—cranial radiation ± intrathecal cytosine arabinoside (meningitis) ± chemotherapy	

Table 26. ***(continued)***

Condition	Treatment	Comment
Dermatologic		
Bacillary angiomatosis	Erythromycin 500 mg po qid × 8 wks	Alternative: Doxycycline, 100 mg bid × 8 wks.
Molluscum contagiosum	Freeze; electrosurgery; curettage, topical cantharidin	
Eosinophilic folliculitis	Astemizole 10 mg qd + topical steroids	Requires constant light
	Ultraviolet light	Efficacy of UV light established (NEJM 1988;318: 1183)
Staphylococcal folliculitis	Cephalexin or dicloxacillin 500 mg po qid × 7–21 days	Add rifampin 600 mg/day × 7 days if severe or refractory Recurrent disease: Chronic antibiotic and/or nasal mupirocin
Dermatophytic fungi	Skin—Topical miconazole or clotrimazole. Refractory cases—griseofulvin, 330–660 mg po/day or ketoconazole, 200 mg po/day × 1–3 mo or itraconazole capsules 100 mg/day. Nails—Griseofulvin, 660 mg/day × 6–15 mo or itraconazole capsules 100–200 mg/day.	Ointments (miconazole and clotrimazole) are over-the-counter
Seborrhea	Skin—Steroid cream (hydrocortisone 1%) or topical ketoconazole applied bid Scalp—shampoos containing zirconium sulfide, salicylic acid or coal tar	Use topical hydrocortisone (2.5%) until lesions resolve, then 1% for maintenance
Gastrointestinal		
Anorexia	Megace, 80 mg po tid or qid	May use up to 800 mg/day. Weight gain is mostly fat.
	Dronabinol (Marinol) 2.5 mg po bid	Synthetic THC, an active ingredient in marijuana. Weight gain is mostly fat.
Nausea/vomiting	Compazine 5–10 mg po q6–8h; Tigan 250 mg po q6–8h; Dramamine 50 mg po q6–8h; Ativan 0.025–0.05 mg/kg IV or IM; Haloperidol, 1–5 mg bid po or IM, Ondansetron (Zofran) 0.2 mg/kg IV or IM	Phenothiazines (Compazine, etc.), haloperidol, benzamides (Tigan, Reglan, etc.) may cause dystonia Must consider medications as cause

Mouth		
Aphthous ulcers	Mouth rinses with Mile's solution, Dexamethasone (0.5 mg/5 ml), dyclonine (10%), Benadryl or viscous Lidocaine (2%)	Miles' solution—60 mg hydrocortisone, 20 cc Mycostatin, 2 gm tetracycline and 120 cc viscous Lidocaine
	Topical fluocinonide (Lidex)	0.05% ointment mixed 1:1 with Orabase and applied 6×/d
	Thalidomide 200 mg po/day/4 wks, then 100 mg 3×/wk Colchicine 1.5 mg/day (J Am Acad Derm 1994; 31:459; Intralesional or topical corticosteroids Prednisone 40 mg/day po × 1–2 wks, then taper (severe or refractory cases)	Thalidomide: initial results are good (Arch Derm 1990;126:923); available through Treatment IND from FDA 301-827-2335.
Oral hairy leukoplakia	Acyclovir 800 mg po 5×/day × 2–3 wks	Most lesions are asymptomatic and do not require treatment; relapses are common when acyclovir is discontinued and may require acyclovir maintenance therapy When treated, most relapse and may require maintenance high-dose acyclovir.
Gingivitis/periodontitis	Metronidazole, 250 mg po tid or 500 mg po bid × 7–14 days, clindamycin, 150–300 mg po qid or amoxicillin-clavulanate 250–500 mg po tid Chlorhexidine gluconate (0.12% as Peridex) for oral rinse bid, topical antiseptic (Betadine) and debridement with curettage	Debridement and curettage is considered essential.
Esophagus		
Candida	Fluconazole 100–200 mg po/d × 14–21 days	Alternatives: Ketoconazole (less effective) (Ann Intern Med 1992;117:655); itraconazole oral solution 100–200 mg/d × 14–21 days (some fluconazole-resistant Candida sp are sensitive) (AAC 1994;38:1530); Amphotericin B (refractory cases).

Table 26. *(continued)*

Condition	Treatment	Comment
Cytomegalovirus	Ganciclovir, 5 mg/kg IV bid × 14–21 days or Foscarnet 60 mg/kg IV q8h × 14–21 days	For patients with complete response, discontinue after induction therapy and use maintenance only if there is relapse
Herpes simplex	Acyclovir, 400–800 mg po 5×/day or 5 mg/kg IV tid × 7–10 days	Relatively rare cause of esophagitis
Aphthous ulcer	Prednisone, 40 mg/day po × 2 wks, then slow taper	
	Thalidomide 200 mg po/d (BMJ 298:432, 1988)	Thalidomide available through Treatment IND 301-827-2335
Diarrhea		
Specific microbial agent		See prior table with listing by specific organism
Bacterial overgrowth	Doxycycline 100 mg po bid, or metronidazole 500–750 mg po bid or amoxicillin-clavulanate 500 mg po qid	Diagnosis requires quantitative culture of small bowel aspirate or hydrogen breath test
Symptomatic treatment	Lomotil/Loperamide/Paregoric, etc.	Utility of bismuth salts (Pepto-Bismol), indomethacin, and octreotide not known
	Diet modification; Frequent small feedings, bland foods, high fiber diet, low fat, no caffeine, no milk or milk products.	
Wasting	Polymeric formulas: Ensure, Sustecal, Enrich, Magnacal, etc.	Polymeric formulas: Non-prescription, about $1.50/can; 10 cans/day required for total caloric needs
	Elemental formulas: Vivonex TEN	Elemental diet for severe malabsorption states; often due to cryptosporidia, less commonly MAC, microsporidia or severe CMV infection; parenteral hyperalimentation rarely used except for cryptosporidiosis with uncontrollable diarrhea.
	Serostim (growth hormone) 6 mg SC qd × 12 wks	Initial study in patients with wasting showed increase in lean body mass and modest weight gain averaging 3 lbs at 12 wks. Cost is $1750/wk

	Thalidomide 100 mg po/day	Potential value ascribed to suppression of TNF; efficacy established for tuberculosis and promising in 3 controlled trials for AIDS patients. Available through Treatment IND: Celgene Co 800-801-8328. Eligibility criterion is weight loss >10% pre-morbid weight
	Megace 400–800 mg/day	Weight gain is mostly fat
	Dronabinol (Marinol) 2.5 mg po bid	Weight gain is mostly fat
	Anabolic steroids	Promotes preservation of muscle mass
	Nandrolone 100–200 mg IM q2 wks	Preferred to testosterone in women
	Testosterone	Often given with megace which is estrogenic
	Testoderm scrotal patch 4 or 6 mg/day	Testosterone is highly androgenic and anabolic; often combined with megace or nandrolone
	Testosterone enanthate or testosterone cypionate, 100–400 IM mg IM q2 wks (usually 200 mg initially)	Testosterone and nandrolone are inexpensive: $2–8/dose q2 wks.
Psychiatric & sleep disorders		
Anxiety	Buspirone (Buspar) 5 mg tid	Nonbenzodiazepine-nonbarbiturate; dependence liability negligible; increase dose 5 mg q2–4 days to effective daily dose of 15–30 mg
Depression	Fluoxetine (Prozac) 10 mg increasing to average 20 mg qd	Major side effects are nausea, nervousness, insomnia, weight loss, dry mouth, constipation; insomnia may be treated with Deseryl 25–50 mg hs
	Nortriptyline (Pamelor) 10–25 mg hs increasing to 50–150 mg hs	Titrate level (70–125 ng/dl); promotes sleep
	Desipramine (Norpramin) 10–25 mg hs increasing to 50–200 mg hs	Titrate level (<125 ng/dl); promotes sleep
	Sertraline (Zoloft) 25–50 mg qd increasing to 50–150 mg/d	Side effects are similar to those noted for Prozac, but less severe due to shorter half-life
Delirium	Haldol (0.5–1 mg) hs	
Insomnia	Diphenhydramine (Benadryl), 25 mg hs	Non-prescription
	Trazodone (Desyrel) 25–50 mg po hs	
	Chloral hydrate 500 mg po hs	Class IV; preferably <1 wk

Table 26. ***(continued)***

Condition	Treatment	Comment
Apathy	Ritalin 5–10 mg tid	
Substance abuse	1. Detoxificiation: sometimes with long-acting benzodiazepines 2. Treatment of co-morbid conditions: mental health (depression, bipolar disorder, schizophrenia, personality disorders, etc.) medical conditions and chronic pain syndromes 3. Maintenance treatment and relapse prevention: individualized to patient need	
Pain (See Medical Letter 1993; 35:1–6) WHO 3 step model	*Step 1* ASA, acetaminophen, 650 mg q4h Nonsteroidal anti-inflammatory agents (Motrin, 200–400 mg q6h; Naprosyn, 250–375 q6–8h; Clinoril 150–200 mg bid, Feldene 10 mg bid *Step 2* Codeine, 30–60 mg q4–6h po SC or IM Oxycodone 5–10 mg po q3–4h Meperidine 50–150 mg q3–4h po, SC, IM, IV *Step 3* Methadone 2.5–10 mg q6–8h po, 10 mg IM Dilaudid 2–4 mg q4–6h po or 3 mg q6–8h by rectal suppositories Morphine 5–20 mg SC, IM, or rectal q4–6h, sustained release 30 mg q12h 20–60 mg po Fentanyl transdermal system 25 mcg/h q72h MS Contin 15–60 mg po bid	Acute pain is best relieved with opioids Chronic pain is best treated with nonopioid initially (ASA, acetaminophen, ibuprofen, nortriptyline) Dependence liability for opioides Side effects of opioides; sedation, constipation, respiratory depression, nausea, and vomiting. Oral codeine, propoxyphene (Darvon), and pentazocine in usual doses are no more effective than ASA. Morphine, Dilaudid, methadone, levorphanol, fentanyl, and large doses of oxycodone are needed for severe pain. Morphine and other full agonists have no limit on analgesic effectiveness except for the limit ascribed to side effects.
Terminal illness	Morphine or other opioides orally or parenterally; MS Contin (continuous release morphine) po 15, 30, 60, or 100 mg; usual dose is 15–60 mg po q12h Patient controlled analgesia (PCA) for morphine Methadone (above doses)	Patients given opioids for acute pain or cancer pain rarely experience euphoria and rarely develop physiologic dependence; clinically significant physical dependence develops after several weeks with large doses

Table 27. Cost of Drugs Commonly Used in Patients with HIV Infection[a]

Drug	Formulation	Typical Regimen	AWP[b] Unit Price ($)	Cost/Wk ($)	Cost/Yr ($)[c]
Acyclovir (Zovirax)	200, 400 mg cap	400 mg po bid	2.11/400 mg cap	29	1,540
	800 mg tab	800 mg po 4–5×/d	4.10/800 mg tab	143	—
	500 mg vial	2 g/d IV	56.60/500 mg vial	1,568	—
Albendazole	200 mg tabs	400–800 mg po bid	0.88/200 mg tab	12–24	—
Alprazolam (Xanax)	0.25, 0.5, 1, & 2 mg tabs	0.25–0.5 mg po bid	0.62/0.25 mg tab	9–18	—
Amikacin (Amikin)	500 mg vial	500 mg bid IV	120/1 g vial	840	—
Amphotericin B	50 mg vial	50 mg/day IV	17.29/50 mg vial	121	—
Amphotericin B Lipid Comlex (Abelcet)	100 mg vial	5 mg/kg/day IV	173/100 mg vial	4,844	—
Amphotericin B (oral)	100 mg/mL	1 mL qid	25.20/24 mL bottle	25	—
Amphotec	100 mg vial	4 mg/kg/day IV	160/100 mg vial	4,480	—
Ampicillin	500 mg cap	500 mg po qid	0.13/500 mg tab	4	—
Ativan (Lorazepam)	1 mg tab	1 mg po bid	0.02/1 mg tab	0.28	—
Atovaquone (Mepron)	750 mg/5 ml	750 mg po bid	538.69/210 mL	179	—
Azithromycin (Zithromax)	250 mg tab	250 mg po qd	6.04/250 mg tab	36	2,184–6,552
	600 mg tab	2 po q wk	14.49/600 mg tab	29	1,508
Benadryl (diphenhydramine)	25 mg cap	25 mg HS	0.18/25 mg cap	1	—
Buspar (Buspirone)	5 mg tab	5 mg po tid	0.62/5 mg tab	11	—
Chlorhexidine (Peridex)		Oral rinse bid	13.93/480 mL bottle	—	—
Cidofovir (Vistide)	375 mg/5 mL	5 mg/kg IV q 2 wk	706.80/375 mg	353	18,356
Ciprofloxacin (Cipro)	250, 500, 750 mg tab	500–750 mg po bid	5.88/750 mg tab	82	—
	400 mg vial	400 mg IV bid	28.80/400 mg vial	400	—
Clarithromycin (Biaxin)	250, 500 mg tab	250–500 mg po bid	3.45/250 mg tab	48	—
			3.45/500 mg tab	48	2,512
Clindamycin (Cleocin)	300 mg cap	300 mg po qid	0.70/150 mg cap	40	—
	300 mg vial	600 mg IV tid	14.58/600 mg vial	306	—
Clotrimazole (Mycelex)	10 mg troche	10 mg po 5×/d	0.82/10 mg troche	28	1,352
d4T (Zerit)	15, 20, 30, 40 mg caps	40 mg bid	3.88/40 mg cap	54	2,800

Table 27. *(continued)*

Drug	Formulation	Typical Regimen	AWP[b] Unit Price ($)	Cost/Wk ($)	Cost/Yr ($)[c]
Dapsone	100 mg tab	100 mg po qd	0.20/100 mg tab	1	65
Deseryl (Trazodone)	50, 100, 150, 300 mg tab	150,400 mg/d	0.12/100 mg tab	1	—
ddI (Videx)	25, 50, 100, 150 mg tab	200 mg po bid	1.53/100 mg tab	42	2,184
ddC (HIVID)	0.375 mg tab 0.75 mg tab	0.75 mg po tid	2.29/0.75 mg tab	42	2,184
Doxycycline	100 mg cap	100 mg po bid	0.11/100 mg tab	1	—
Dronabinol (Marinol)	2.5, 5 mg	2.5 mg po bid	2.98/2.5 mg	42	2,184
Erythromycin	250 mg cap	500 mg po qid	0.14/250 mg cap	4	—
Erythropoietin (Procrit, Epogen)	2000, 3000, 4000 unit vials	30,000 U 3×/wk	36/3000 U vial (12/1000 U)	1,080	—
Ethambutol	400 mg tab	400 mg po tid	1.72/400 mg tab	36	1,878
Feeding supplements Ensure Sustecal, etc.	240 mL	240 mL ×4/d	1.50/240 mL	42	1,460
Vivonex TEN	1 packet	4 packets/d	6.08/packet	170	8,840
Fentanyll patch	25, 50, 75, 100 μg/hr	25 μg/hr q 72 h	10/25 μg/hr	30	—
Fluconazole (Diflucan)	50 mg	50 mg po qd	4.38/50 mg tab	30	1,560
	100 mg	100 mg po bid	6.88/100 mg tab	96	4,992
	400 mg vial	200 mg IV bid	118.67/400 mg vial	830	—
Fluoxetine (Prozac)	10, 20 mg caps	10–40 mg/day	2.34/20 mg cap	31–62	—
Flurazepam (Dalmane)	15, 30 mg caps	15–30 mg hs	0.06/30 mg cap	1	—
Foscarnet (Foscavir)	6, 12 gm vial	6 g IV qd	73.25/6 g vial	513	26,690
Gammaglobulin (Gamimune, etc.)	250 mL vial 5%	60 g IV	714/250 mL vial	3,570/dose	—
Ganciclovir (Cytovene)	500 mg vial	350 mg IV qd	34.80/500 mg vial	170	8,800
Ganciclovir oral	250 mg caps	1 g po tid	3.90/250 mg tab	327	—
G-CSF (Filgrastim, Neupogen)	300, 480 μg vial	75–300 μg IV or SC qd or qod	156.10/300 μg vial	133–1,066	—
Growth hormone (Serostim)	6 mg vial	6 mg SC/d	42/6 mg vial	1,750	—
Halcion (Triazolam)	0.125, 0.25 mg tab	0.25 mg HS	0.78/0.25 mg tab	5	—

Haloperidol (Haldol)	1 mg tab	2 mg bid	0.55/1 mg tab	2	—
Hepatitis B vaccine	10, 20 μg/mL	1 mL SC ×3	156/3 doses	—	160
Interferon-α (Roferon)	3 mil U vial	3–30 mil U IV or SC qd	32.94/3 mil U vial	220–2,200	—
Isoniazid (INH)	300 mg tab	300 mg po qd	0.02/300 mg tab	0.14	50
Itraconazole (Sporanox)	100 mg capsule	100 mg po bid	5.60/100 mg tab	78	3,900
	100 mg/10 ml oral solution	100 mg/d	6.88/100 mg		
Indinavir	200, 400 mg caps	800 mg tid	2.50/400 mg cap	105	5,460
Ketoconazole (Nizoral)	200 mg tab	200 mg po qd	2.82/200 mg tab	20	1,040
Lamivudine (3TC, Epivir)	150 mg tabs	150 mg bid	3.84/150 mg tab	54	2,795
Leucovorin (Folinic acid)	5, 10, 15, 25 mg tabs	10 mg po qd	2.95/5 mg tab	40	2,080
			21/25 mg tab		
Levofloxacin (Levaquin)	250, 500 mg tabs	500 mg po qd	7.00/500 mg		
		500 mg IV qd	39.50/500 mg		
Lomotil	2.5 mg tab	5 mg po qid	0.50/2.5 mg tab	18	—
Loperamide (Imodium)	2 mg cap	2 mg 6×/d	0.65/2 mg	27	—
Megace	20, 40 mg tab	80 mg po qid	1.29/40 mg	72	3,588
Methadone	5, 10 mg tab	15–40 mg/d	0.14/10 mg tab	2–3	—
Metronidazole	250, 500 mg tab	250 mg po tid	0.03/250 mg tab	<1	—
	500 mg vial	.5–1 gm IV bid	7.81/500 mg vial	8–56	—
Morphine sulfate (MS contin)	30 mg tab		1.32/30 mg tab		
Nelfinavir (Viracept)	250 mg tab	750 mg tid	1.75/250 mg tab	110	5720
Nevirapine (Viramune)	200 mg tabs	200 mg po bid	4.13/200 mg tab		
Nortriptyline (Pamelor)	10, 25, 50 mg cap	75 mg po HS	0.24/75 mg caps	2	—
Nystatin	100,000 units/mL	5 HTU po 5×/d	0.26/5 mL	9	468
Octreotide (Sandostatin)	50, 100, 200, 500, 1,000 μg/m L vial	100–500 μg SC tid	102.60/1 mg vial		
Ofloxacin (Floxin)	400 mg tab	400 mg po bid	3.98/400 mg tab	56	—
	400 mg vial	400 mg IV bid	26.40/400 mg vial	370	—
Paromomycin	250 mg caps	500–750 mg po qid	2.07/250 mg cap	173	—

Table 27. ***(continued)***

Drug	Formulation	Typical Regimen	AWP[b] Unit Price ($)	Cost/Wk ($)	Cost/Yr ($)[c]
Pentamidine	300 mg vial	300 mg aerosolized	98.75/300 mg	25	1,200
		300 mg IV qd	98.75/300 mg	691	—
Pneumovax	0.5 mL vial	0.5 mL × 1	10.60/0.5 mL	—	11
Prednisone	50 mg tab	50 mg po qd	0.16/50 mg tab	2	—
Primaquine	15 mg tab	15 mg/d	0.64/15 mg tab	5	—
Prozac (Fluoxetine)	10, 20 mg parv	10–40 mg po qd	2.34/20 mg parvule	16–32	—
Pyrazinamide	500 mg tab	500 mg po qid	1.12/500 mg tab	31	1,612
Pyrimethamine (Daraprim)	25 mg tab	50 mg po qd	0.41/25 mg tab	5	260
Retrovir (AZT Zidovudine)	100 mg cap	200 mg po tid	1.55/100 mg cap	65	2,905
			3.98/300 mg tab		
Rifabutin (Mycobutin)	150 mg cap	300 mg po qd	3.87/150 mg cap	54	2,817
Rifampin	300 mg cap	600 mg po qd	1.61/300 mg cap	23	1,196
Rifater	50 mg INH, 120 mg Rif, 300 mg PZA	1 tab/10 kg/d	1.80/tab	75	—
Ritalin	10 mg tab	10 mg po tid	0.40/10 mg tab	8	—
Ritonavir	100 mg cap	600 mg bid	1.85/100 mg cap	155	8,103
Saquinavir	200 mg tabs	600 mg po tid	2.12/200 mg cap	133	6,945
Serostim	5 mg vials	6 mg/day IM	42/mg	1,750	—
Sulfadiazine	500 mg tab	.5–2 gm qid	0.55/500 mg tab	3	—
Testosterone	100–400 mg IM	20.65/200 mg vial		2	—
Trimethoprim	100, 200 mg tabs	300 mg tid	0.25/200 mg tab	10	—
Trimethoprim-sulfamethoxazole	SS tab	1 DS po qd	0.07/DS tab	1	30
	DS tab	2 DS po tid		3	—
		16/80 mg/mL vial	3.53/10 mL vial	100	—
Trimetrexate (Neutrexin)	25 mg vials puvule	45 mg/m^2 IV/d	60.84/25 mg vial	1,703	—
Vancomycin	125 mg puvule	125 mg po qid	5.10/125 mg		—
	0.5, 1 gm vial	1 g bid IV	7.80/500 mg vial		
Vivonex TEN	1 packet	4 packs po qd	6.20/packet	173	8,996
Xanax (Aprazolam)	0.25, 0.5, 1, 2 mg	0.25 mg po bid	.62/0.25 mg tab	8	437

[a] Average wholesale prices from Medispan, Hospital Formulary Pricing Guide, January 1997.
[b] AWP, average wholesale price.
[c] Annual costs are approximate AWP and restricted to drugs given chronically.

Table 28. Adverse Reactions (by Class) to Antimicrobial Agents Commonly Used in Patients with HIV Infection

	Frequent	Occasional	Rare
Acyclovir	Irritation at infusion site (IV infusion)	Nausea and vomiting; diarrhea	CNS toxicity with agitation, encephalopathy, disorientation, seizures; hallucinations; anemia; neutropenia; thrombocytopenia; hypotension; rash; renal toxicity especially with prior renal disease; hepatotoxicity; pruritis
Albendazole (Eskazole)		Hepatotoxity, reversible neutropenia—monitor CBC and liver function tests	
Aminoglycosides Tobramycin Gentamicin Amikacin Netilmicin Kanamycin	Renal failure-dose related; monitor creatinine ≥ 3×/wk	Vestibular and auditory toxicity—dose related	Fever; rash; blurred vision; neuromuscular blockage; eosinophilia
Aminosalicylic acid (PAS)	GI intolerance	Liver damage; allergic reactions; thyroid enlargement	Acidosis; vasculitis; hypoglycemia (diabetes); hypokalemial encephalopathy; decreased prothrombin activity; myalgias; renal damage; gastric hemorrhage
Amphotericin B	Fever (maximal at 1 hr) and chills (at 2 hrs) (Prevent/reduce with hydrocortisone, ibuprophen, ASA, acetaminophen, meperidine); renal	Nausea, vomiting; metallic taste; headache; phlebitis at infusion site	Hypotension; rash; pruritus; blurred vision; peripheral neuropathy; convulsions; hemorrhagic gastroenteritis;

Amphotericin B lipid complex—comparisons

Side effect	Ampho B	Abelcet	Amphotec
Chills/fever	40–50%	15–20%	50–70%
Creatinine rise	30–40%	10%	10–20%
Hypotension	5–10%	5–10%	5–10%
Hypokalemia	20%	5%	10%

Table 28. ***(continued)***

	Frequent	Occasional	Rare
	damage—dose dependent and reversible in absence of prior renal damage and dose <3 gm; reduce with hydration and sodium supplementation; low K^+ and Mg^{++}; anemia		Diabetes insipidus; pulmonary edema; anaphylaxis; acute hepatic failure; eosinophilia; leukopenia; thrombocytopenia
Atovaquone (Mepron)	Rash (20%), nausea (20%), diarrhea (20%); these are sufficiently severe to require discontinuation in 9%	Vomiting, pruritis	Headache, fever, insomnia
Azithromycin		GI intolerance (dose related) (6%); diarrhea (4%), reversible ototoxicity (2%), skin rash (1%), headache, fatigue, drowsiness (1%)	Erythema multiforme; increased transaminase Pseudomembranous colitis
Benzodiazepines	Dependency, tolerance, and withdrawal reactions (related to dose and duration); daytime sedation, dizziness, ataxia	Blurred vision, diplopia, confusion, memory disturbance amnesia, fatigue, incontinence, constipation, hypotension, bizarre behavior	
Buspirone	CNS: dizziness, headache, sedation (10%), warn patient	Psychomotor dysfunction, fatigue, anxiety, insomnia (5%); nausea (6–8%); depression (3%); dream disturbance; GI: dry mouth, constipation, diarrhea (1–5%); tachycardia (2%); sexual dysfunction	
Capreomycin	Renal damage (tubular necrosis esp. in patients with prior renal damage): Increased creatinine, proteinuria, cylindruria; monitor UA and creatinine weekly	Ototoxicity (vestibular > auditory) should assess vestibular function before and during treatment; electrolyte abnormalities; pain, induration and sterile abscesses at injection sites	Allergic reactions; leukopenia; leukocytosis; neuromuscular blockage (large IV doses—reversed with neostigmine); hypersensitivity reactions; hepatitis?

Cephalosporins	Phlebitis at infusion sites; diarrhea (esp. cefoperazone); pain at IM injection sites (less with cefazolin)	Allergic reactions (anaphylaxis rare); diarrhea and colitis including C. difficile-associated colitis and PMC; hypoprothrombinemia (cefamandole, cefoperazone, moxalactam, cefmetazole and cefotetan); eosinophilia; positive Coombs' test	Hemolytic anemia; interstitial nephritis (cephalothin); hepatic dysfunction; convulsions (high dose with renal failure); neutropenia; thrombocytopenia
Cidofovir	Renal failure—25% develop ≥ 2+ proteinuria or creatinine increase >2–3 mg/dL (reversible if discontinued). Most give IV hydration and probenecid. Probenecid side effects in 50%: fever, rash, headache, nausea, GI intolerance—reduce	Neutropenia in 15%, Fanconi syndrome	
Ciprofloxacin (See quinolones)			
Clarithromycin (Biaxin)		GI intolerance (4%), headache (2%); antibiotic-associated diarrhea, transaminase elevation	Rare
Clindamycin (Cleocin)	Diarrhea (10–30%)	Nausea, vomiting, anorexia morbilliform rash, pruritis C. difficile-associated colitis or PMC	Stevens-Johnson syndrome; joint pains; neutropenia; thrombocytopenia
Clotrimazole		Oral—increased transaminase (15%), nausea and vomiting (5%) Topical (skin and vaginal): rash, burning	

Table 28. ***(continued)***

	Frequent	Occasional	Rare
Cycloserine	CNS: anxiety, confusion, depression, somnolence, disorientation, headache, hallucinations, tremor, hyperreflexia, increased CSF protein and pressure (dose related and reversible); contraindicated in active alcoholics; twitching and seizures prevented with large doses of pyridoxine (100 mg tid)	Liver damage; malabsorption; peripheral neuropathy; folate deficiency; anemia	Coma: seizures (contraindicated in epileptics); hypersensitivity reactions; heart failure, arrhythmias
d4T (Stavudine)(Zerit)	Perpheral neuropathy (19–24%)—Reduce dose to 20 mg bid or discontinue	Pancreatitis (0.5–1%); headache; GI intolerance	Neutropenia
Dapsone	Rash, fever, nausea, anorexia, neutropenia—sufficiently severe to require discontinuation in 30–40%; Hemolytic anemia (dose dependent)	Blood dyscrasias: methemoglobulinemia and sulfahemoglobinemia ± G-6-PD deficiency; allergic reactions; insomnia; irritability; headache (transient) blurred vision, ringing in ears; hepatitis	Hypoalbuminema; epidermal necrolysis; optic atrophy; aplastic anemia; agranulocytosis; peripheral neuropathy; aplastic anemia; ``sulfone syndrome''—fever, exfoliative dermatitis, jaundice, adenopathy, methemoglobinemia and anemia—treat with steroids; nephrosis
Daunorubicin	Granulocytopenia—monitor CBC predose Triad of flushing, back pain, and chest tightness-14%; follows infusions and resolves with discontinuation or slowing of infusion	Cardiotoxicity especially with prior cardiac disease or prior treatment with anthracyclines. Monitor ejection fraction with use of large doses (≥320 mg/m^2)	Extravasation—tissue necrosis

Didanosine (ddl; Videx)	Diarrhea (15–30%) Pancreatitis (1–9%)—risk is increased with history of pancreatitis, alcoholism, late-stage HIV; some monitor anylase levels Peripheral neuropathy (painful feet, dose related 5–12%)—reduce dose or discontinue Note: Na^{++} load of 265 mg/tab and 1350 mg/powder packet	Nausea; vomiting; rash; neutropenia; headache; hyperuricemia; hepatitis (3–17%)	Cardiomyopathy; Lactic acidosis, steatotosis syndrome (?)
Dideoxycytidine (ddC; HIVID)	Peripheral neuropathy 17–31%; frequency is related to cumulative dose; flu-like complaints	Aphthous ulcers; rash; pancreatitis (<1%); hepatitis	Thrombocytopenia; leukopenia; lactic acidosis-steatotosis syndrome (?) cardiomyopathy
Doxycycline	Gi intolerance (10%), photosensitivity; diarrhea (reduced with food); Candida vaginitis		
Dronabinol (Marinol)	Dose related mood high somnolence, confusion (usually resolves with continued use in 1–3 days)	Abuse potential, esp. with substance abusers, elderly patients with psychiatric illness and those receiving sedatives, hypnotics, etc.	
EPO (epogen, Procrit)		Headache; arthralgias, flu-like illness, GI intolerance, diarrhea fatigue	Hypertension, seizures (?)
Erythromycins	GI intolerance (oral-dose related); phlebitis (IV)	Diarrhea; stomatitis; cholestatic hepatitis (esp. estolate-	Allergic reactions; colitis; hemolytic anemia;

Table 28. ***(continued)***

	Frequent	Occasional	Rare
		reversible); generalized rash	reversible ototoxicity (esp. with high doses and renal failure)
Erythropoeitin		Headache; arthralgias (seizures and hypertension in renal dialysis patients, but not AIDS patients)	
Ethambutol		Optic neuritis: decreased acuity, reduced color discrimination, constricted fields, scotomata—dose related and infrequent with 15 mg/kg/day	Hypersensitivity; peripheral neuropathy; thrombocytopenia; toxic epidermal neurolysis; lichenoid skin rash
Ethionamide	GI intolerance (CNS effect)	Allergic reactions; peripheral neuropathy (prevented with pyridoxine); reversible liver damage (9%) with jaundice (1–3%)—monitor transaminase q 2–4 wk	Optic neuritis; gouty arthritis; hypothyroidism; impotence; hypothyroidism; purpura; poor diabetic control; rash
Fentanyl patch		Central nervous system depression and respiratory depression—especially in opiate-naive patients; dose related Tolerance with extended courses Local side effects: erythema, pruritis, edema at site of application	
Fluconazole		GI intolerance (1.5–8%); rash (5%); transient increased in transaminase (5%) elevation to ≥8× normal (1%); headache	Hepatitis; Stevens-Johnson syndrome; thrombocytopenia; anaphylaxis; hypokalemia

		(2%); diarrhea; prolonged protime with coumadin; reversible alopecia)(10–20%) with ≥400 mg/day at median of 3 mo after starting (Ann Intern Med 123:354, 1995)	
Flucytosine	GI intolerance (including nausea, vomiting, diarrhea, and ulcer-active colitis)	Marrow suppression with leukopenia or thrombocytopenia (dose related, esp. with renal failure, level >100 mcg/mL, or concurrent amphotericin); confusion; rash; hepatitis (dose related)	Hallucinations; eosinophilia; granulocytosis; fatal hepatitis; -eripheral neuropathy
Fluoxetine (Prozac)	GI intolerance (20%); anxiety, agitation insomnia (20%)	Headache, tremor, drowsiness, dry mouth, sweating, diarrhea, sexual dysfunction, skin rash	Acute dystonia, akathisia
Foscarnet	Renal failure (usually reversible)—30% get creatininte >2 mg/dL (monitor creatinine 1–3×/week and discontinue if creatinine clearance <0.4 mL/min/kg or creatinine >2.9 mg/dL)	Mineral and electrolyte changes:—reduced Ca^{++}, ionized Ca^{++}, Mg^{++}, PO_4^-, K^+ (8–16%) (monitor electrolytes 1–2×/wk and symptoms—parasthesias, and numbness); ionized calcium, seizures (10%); penile ulcers; nausea-relieved with slowing infusion or anti-nausea agent	
G-CSF (Neupogen) (Figrastim)	Bone pain in 10–20% (usually controlled with acetaminiophen)	Erythema or pain at injection site	Anemia, thrombocytopenia, wheezing, acute febrile dermatosis (Sweet's syndrome); Vasculitis
Ganciclovir (DHPG) (Cytovene)	Neutropenia with absolute neutrophil count <1000/mL in 25–50% (monitor CBC 2–3×/wk and discontinue if ANC <500/mm^3 or platelet count <25,000/mm^3); dose related and reversible in 3–7 days after	Thrombocytopenia (2–8%); Anemia (2%); fever; rash; changes in mental status; abnormal liver function tests (2%); CNS toxicity with headache, seizures, confusion, coma (10–15%); GI	Psychosis; neuropathy; impaired reproductive function (?); hematuria; renal failure; nausea; vomiting; GI bleeding or perforation; myocardiopathy;

Table 28. ***(continued)***

	Frequent	Occasional	Rare
	discontinuation or with treatment using G-CSF or GM-CSF	intolerance (2%)	hypotension; ataxia; coma; somnolence
Ganciclovir, oral	Neutropenia with ANC <500/mL in 18%; anemia with Hgb <8 in 10%; monitor CBC ± treatment	Renal failure (creatinine >2.5 mg/dL in 4%)	
Haloperidol (Haldol)	CNS: Extrapyramidal symptoms	CNS: Dystonia, motor restlessness; tardive dyskinesia (abrupt withdrawal); sexual dysfunction (10–20%)	Neuroleptic malignant syndrome; hypotension; hepatitis
Ibuprofen	GI intolerance (give with milk); increased transaminase levels—15%	Peptic ulcer: bleed or perforation; CNS—dizziness, headache, anxiety; tinnitis	Aseptic meningitis amblyopia, hearing loss; severe liver toxicity; marrow suppression; renal failure; anaphylaxis
Interferon-α	Flu-like (80% with 35 mil units/d): fever, fatigue, anorexia, headache, myalgias, depression; Reduce with NSAIDS; GI intolerance (20–65%); nausea, vomiting, abdominal pain, diarrhea	CNS toxicity: Confusion, paresthias, concentration problems; amnesia; pruritis; marrow supression; alopecia; proteinuria	Delirium, obtundation
Indinavir	Asymptomatic increase in indirect bilirubia (10–15%)	Nephrolithiasis 5–15%—must take ≥48 oz fluids/d; dry skin and lips; GI intolerance—nausea, vomiting	Metalic taste, fatique, insomnia, blurred vision, dizziness, rash, thrombocytopenia
Isoniazid	Hepatitis—age related <20 yrs, nil; 35, 6%; 45, 11%; 55, 18%; patient should be warned of symptoms and drug should be discontinued if transaminase levels are 3× normal limit	Allergic reactions; fever; peripheral neuropathy reduce with pyridoxine (25–50 mg/d) which is advocated with alcoholism, diabetes, pregnancy, or malnutrition	CNS—optic neuritis; psychosis; convulsions; toxic encephalopathy; twitching; coma; blood dyscrasias; hyperglycemia; lupus-like syndrome; keratitis; pellagra-like rash

Itraconazole (Sporanox)	GI intolerance (5–10%); rash (8%); treatment discontinued in 10%	Pruritis; headaches; asthenia; diarrhea; dizziness; hepatitis (2–3%); importence (1%)	Fulminant hepatitis (1:1000 and reversible)
Ketoconazole	GI intolerance (dose related); temporary increase in transaminase levels (2–5%)	Endocrine—decreased steroid and testosterone synthesis with impotence, gynecomastia, oligospermia, reduced libido; menstrual abnormalities (prolonged use and dose related, usually ≥600 mg/d); headache; dizziness; asthenia; pruritis; rash	Abrupt hepatitis (1:15,000); rare cases of fatal hepatic necrosis; anaphylaxis; lethargy; arthralgias; fever; marrow suppression; hypothyroidism (genetically determined); thrombocytopenia; hallucinations
Lamivudine (3TC) (Epivir)		Headache, nausea, diarrhea, abdominal pain, insomnia	
Levofloxacin (Levoquin)—see Quinolones			
Megesterol acetate (Megace)		Sexual dysfunction (estrogen—may respond to testosterone); diarrhea; rash; asthenia; flatulence; pain; GI intolerance; hyperglycemia (5%)	Carpal tunnel syndrome, thrombosis, vaginal bleeding, alopecia, high dose (480–1600 mg/d)—chest pressure, hypertension, dyspnea, congestive heart failure
Metronidazole (Flagyl)	GI intolerance; metallic taste; headache	Peripheral neuropathy (prolonged use, reversible—usually reversible); phlebitis at injection sites; Antabuse-like reaction with alcohol ingestion	Seizures; ataxic encephalitis; colitis; leukopenia; dysuria; pancreatitis; allergic reactions; mutagenic in Ames test (clinical relevance as carcinogen with long-term use is unclear)

Table 28. ***(continued)***

	Frequent	Occasional	Rare
Morphine + other opiate agonists	Tolerance, physical dependence, psychological dependence, withdrawal syndrome (slight with 80 mg MS/d × 30 d; severe with 240 mg MS/d × 30 d)	Acute toxicity: coma, respiratory depression, cardiac arrest	
Nelfinavir (Viracept)		Diarrhea—10% sufficiently severe to require discontinuation in 1.6%	
Nevirapine (Viramune)	Rash—17%—usually maculopapular and erythematous ± pruritis; discontinue if rash is severe, accompanied by fever, blisters, or mucous membrane involvement	Hepatitis; nausea	Fever, headache
Nortriptyline and other tricyclics (Pamelor, Aventyl)	Anticholinergic activity: dry mucous membranes, blurred vision, constipation, urinary retention; CNS: drowsiness, weakness, fatigue	Extrapyramidal symptoms: tremor, rigidity, dystonia, dysarthria; increased transaminase levels; weight gain; sexual dysfunction orthostatic hypotension	Neuroleptic malignant syndrome, peripheral neuropathy, ataxia, marrow suppression; hepatitis; arrhythmias
Nystatin		GI intolerance	
Octreotide (Sandostatin)	Cholelithiasis or biliary sludge (15%); GI intolerance—nausea, vomiting, cramping, diarrhea (5–15%)	Headache, dizziness, lightheadedness, asthenia (1–2%); hypoglycemia (1–2%)	
Paromomycin (Humatin)		GI intolerance, steatorrhea and malabsorption	Rash, headache, vertigo Aminoglycoside: With GI absorption ± renal failure, there could be nephrotoxicity or ototoxicity

Penicillins	Hypersensitivity reactions; rash (esp. ampicillin and amoxicillin); diarrhea (esp. ampicillin, amoxicillin and nafcillin)	GI intolerance (oral agents); fever; Coombs' test positive; phlebitis at infusion sites and sterile abscesses at IM sites; Jarisch-Herxheimer reaction (syphilis or other spirochetal infections)	Anaphylaxis; leukopenia thrombocytopenia; colitis (esp. ampicillin)l hepatic damage; renal damage; CNS—seizures; twitching (high doses in patients with renal failure); hyperkalemia (penicillin G infusion); abnormal platelet aggregation with bleeding diathesis (carbenicillin and ticarcillin)
Pentamidine	Nephrotoxicity (25%); usually second week of treatment and usually reversible; IM injection: pain, tenderness, and induration (10–20%)	Hypotension (esp. with rapid infusions); hypoglycemia (5–10%), usually after 1 wk, may last days with glucose <25 mg/dL; hyperglycemia and insulin-dependent diabetes; GI intolerance: nausea, vomiting, abdominal pain, anorexia and/or bad taste; marrow suppression with leukopenia or thrombocytopenia	Hepatotoxicity; leukopenia; thrombocytopenia; pancreatitis; hypocalcemia; rash, pruritis, fever, urticaria; anaphylaxis; toxic epidermal necrolysis
	Aerosolized administration—cough (30%—prevent with Albuterol, 2 puffs)	Aerosol administration—asthma reaction (5%—prevent with Albuterol, 2 puffs), laryngitis, chest pain	

Table 28. ***(continued)***

	Frequent	Occasional	Rare
Phenytoin (Dilantin)	Blood levels >25 mcg/mL; nystagmus, ataxia, diplopia; >30 mcg/mL: lethargy; >50: extreme lethargy	GI intolerance; gingival hypertrophy; rash; fever; lymphadenopathy. Blood levels >25 mcg/mL: IV infusion: hypotension, vein irritation, inflammation with extravasation; sexual dysfunction; hepatitis; lab tests: protime increased, pos LE prep, glucose increased, calcium decreased, thyroid hormones—T3 & T4—increased.	Dyskinesias; marrow suppression; periarteritis nodosa; acute psychosis
Primaquine		Hemolytic anemia (G-6-PD deficiency warn patient to observe for dark urine and/or screen with G-6-PD level pretreatment; GI intolerance (give with meals)	Headache; pruritis Methemoglobinemia, hypertension, arrhythmias, disturbed visual accommodation
Pyrazinamide	Nongouty polyarthralgia; asymptomatic hyperuricemia	Hepatitis (dose related, frequency not increased when given with INH or rifampin, rarely serious); syndrome of hepatomegaly, fever, and anorexia; GI intolerance; gout (treat with allopurinol or probenecid)	Rash; fever; porphyria; photosensitivity; acute yellow atrophy of liver; acne; skin discoloration; pruritis; sideroblastic anemia; thrombocytopenia
Pyrimethamine		Folic acid deficiency with megaloblastic anemia and pancytopenia (dose related and reversed with leucovorin);	CNS—ataxia, tremors, seizures (dose related), fatigue, headache, depression, insomnia

		allergic reactions (primarily with Fansidar); GI intolerance (reduce dose or give with meals)	
Quinolones	(Animal studies show arthropathies in weight-bearing joints of immature animals; significance in humans is not known, but this class is considered contraindicated in children and during pregnancy)	GI intolerance (1–5%); CNS—headache, malaise, insomnia, dizziness; allergic reactions: rash (mild and transient in 1–4%); Candida vaginitis; tendon rupture—25 reported cases; photosensitivity—sparfloxacin (8%)	Papilledema; nystagmus; visual disturbances; diarrhea; PMC; abnormal liver function tests including hepatic necrosis; marrow suppression; photosensitivity; anaphylaxis; seizures; toxic psychosis; CNS stimulation—tremors, restlessness, confusion, arthralgias; interstitial nephritis, renal failure
Retrovir (AZT, Zidovudine)	Marrow suppression with anemia or leukopenia related to dose, stage of disease and duration of treatment; reversible with discontinuation and/or G-CSF or EPO. Monitor CBC and discontinue with Hgb <8 g/dL or ANC < 750/dL. Macrocytosis—not considered a side effect, but useful for monitoring compliance	Subjective complaints with headache, flu-like symptoms, insomnia and/or myalgias—dose related; myopathy with extremity weakness and elevated CPK—reversible with discontinuation); nail pigmentation; GI intolerance—esp nausea	Seizures (reversible); allergy (rash, anaphylaxis); twitching; mania; hepatitis; cardiomyopathy (ECHO shows decrease EF); Lactic acidosis—steatosis syndrome
Rifabutin (Mycobutin)	Note: Uveitis is a dose-related complication seen with >300 mg/day and/or concurrent clarithromycin, indinavir, ritonavir, saquinavir, or flucoconazole. Presentation is a red, painful eye with blurring, photophobia, or floaters. Most	Hepatitis; rash (4–10%), leukopenia (3%), thrombocytopenia (usually mild and transient); GI intolerance (5–10%); flu-like illness with interrupted treatment; drug interactions identical to rifampin; dose-	Dose-related polyarthralgias; thrombotic thrombocytopenic purpura; hemolysis; myositis; confusion; seizures

Table 28. ***(continued)***

	Frequent	Occasional	Rare
	respond to topical steroids + mydriatrics (NEJM 330:438, 1994)	related pseudojuandice with yellow skin pigmentation, without scleral icterus or elevated bilirubin	
Rifampin	Orange discoloration of urine, tears (contact lens), sweat	Hepatitis (cholestatic changes usually in the first month of treatment—frequency not increased when given with INH); jaundice (usually reversible with dose reduction and/or continued use); GI intolerance; hypersensitivity reactions (esp. with intermittent use); CNS: headache, fatigue, confusion, especially in first weeks of treatment; induces cytochrome P450 to reduce drug levels (see drug interactions); flu-like symptoms with intermittent use characterized by fever, aches ± dyspnea, wheezing	Thrombocytopenia; leukopenia; eosinophilia; hemolytic anemia; renal damage; proximal myopathy; hyperuricemia; anaphylaxis
Ritonavir	GI intolerance, increase cholesterol and triglycerides, Extensive drug interactions	Circumoral and peripheral paresthesias	
Saquinavir		GI intolerance: nausea, diarrhea, abdominal pain	Headache; hepatitis; thrombocytopenia, rash, allergic reaction
Serostim (growth hormone)		Fluid and sodium retention with edema, arthralgias, and hypertension; musculoskeletal discomfort (20–50%) with increased tissue turgor and swelling of hands and feet	Flu-like symptoms, rigors, back pain, malaise, carpal tunnel syndrome, chest pain, nausea, diarrhea

Stavudine (d4T)	Peripheral neuropathy (15–21%), dose related	Pancreatitis (0.5–1%)	Hepatotoxicity, granulocytopenia
Sulfonamides	Rash, pruritis, fever, leukopenia	Erythema multiforme, Stevens-Johnson syndrome, serum sickness; crystalluria with renal damage, urolithiasis and oliguria—dose related and prevented with high output or alkaline urine; GI intolerance; hepatitis	Myocarditis; psychosis; neuropathy; dizziness; depression; hemolytic anemia (G-6-PD deficiency); marrow suppression; agranulocytosis; photosensitivity
Testosterone (IM)	Androgenic (and anabolic) effects—acne, flushing, virilizing to women, gynecomastia, increased libido, priapism, edema	Cholestatic hepatitis	
Tetracyclines	GI intolerance (dose related); stains and deforms teeth in children <8 yrs; vertigo (minocycline); negative nitrogen balance and increased axotemia with renal failure (except doxycycline); vaginitis	Hepatotoxicity (dose related, esp. IV use in pregnant women); esophageal ulcerations; diarrhea; candidiasis (thrush and vaginitis); photosensitivity (esp. demeclocycline); phlebitis with IV treatment and pain with IM injection	Malabsorptions; allergic reactions; visual disturbances; aggravation of myasthenia; hemolytic anemia; colitis
Trazodone (Desyrel)	Sedation in 15–20%	Orthostatic hypotension (5%) Anticholinergic effects—less compared with tricyclics Nervousness, fatigue, dizziness, agitation	Priapism (1/6000)
Trimethoprim	Hyperkalemia in 20–50% given >15 mg/kg/day (NEJM 328: 703, 1993); GI intolerance (dose related)	Marrow: megaloblastic anemia, neutropenia, thrombocytopenia; rash (3%)	Pancytopenia

Table 28. *(continued)*

	Frequent	Occasional	Rare
Trimethoprim-sulfamethoxazole (Bactrim, Septra)	Fever, leukopenia, pruritis, rash (AIDS patients: 30–40% required discontinuation, but 60–70% tolerate the drug with readministration; dose related)	GI intolerance: nausea, vomiting, anorexia, diarrheal Candida vaginitis; hepatitis including cholestatic jaundice; anemia; thrombocytopenia renal failure, thema multiforme, Stevens-Johnson syndrome; anemia; thrombocytopenia	Ataxis, apathy, ankle clonus, hemolytic anemia due to G-6-PD deficiency Steven-Johnson syndrome, erythema multiforme; *C. difficile* associated colitis or PMC; pancreatitis; hepatic necrosis
Trimetrexate (Neutrexin)	Bone marrow suppression—must add leucovorin (thrombocytopenia and neutropenia)	Oral or GI ulceration renal dysfunction, hepatotoxicity	
Vancomycin	Phlebitis at injection site	''Red-man syndrome'': flushing ± dyspnea, urticaria, pruritis, and/or wheezing ascribed to histamine release and directly related to rate of infusion—treat with slowing infusion ± antihistamines, corticosteroids, and/or IV fluids; eosinophilia; allergic reactions with rash; promotes nephrotoxicity and ototoxicity of other drugs esp. aminoglycosides	Anaphylaxis; ototoxicity and ? nephrotoxicity (dose related); peripheral neuropathy; marrow suppression

Table 29. Drug Interactions

Drug	Effect of Interaction
Acyclovir	
Narcotics	Increased meperidine levels
Probenecid	Increased acyclovir levels
Amphotericin B	
Aminoglycosides	Increased nephrotoxicity[a]
Capreomycin	Increased nephrotoxicity[a]
Corticosteroids	Increased hypokalemia
Cisplatin	Increased nephrotoxicity
Cyclosporine	Increased nephrotoxicity
Digitalis	Increased cardiotoxicity (monitor K^+)
Diuretics	Increased hypokalemia
Methoxyflurane	Increased nephrotoxicity
Skeletal muscle relaxants	Increased effect of relaxants
Vancomycin	Increased nephrotoxicity
Atovaquone	
AZT	Increased AZT levels (significance is ?)
Food (fat)	Increased absorption—*should be taken with meals*
Rifampin and rifabutin	Decreased atovaquone levels[a]
Azithromycin	
Antacids with Al^{++} or Mg^{++}	Decreased absorption
Coumadin	Increased prothrombin time
Food	Decreased absorption
Theophylline	Increased theophylline levels
AZT (Retrovir, Zidovudine)	
Amphotericin B	Increased anemia
Atovaquone	Increased AZT levels
Cancer chemotherapy (adriamycin, vinblastine, vincristine)	Increased marrow toxicity
Clarithromycin	Decreased AZT absorption, give ≥2 hr apart
d4T (Stavudine)	Antagonistic vs. HIV
Dapsone	Increased marrow toxicity
Fluconazole (400 mg/d)	Increased AZT levels
Flucytosine	Increased leukopenia
Ganciclovir	Increased leukopenia, concurrent use contraindicated except with G-CSF[a]
Interferon	Increased leukopenia
Phenytoin	Decreased phenytoin levels
Probenecid	Increased AZT levels (and rash)
Benzodiazepines	
Caffeine	Antagonizes sedative effect
Cimetidine	Increase benzodiazepine toxicity
Erythromycin	Increase benzodiazepine toxicity
Isoniazid	Increase benzodiazepine toxicity
Omeprazole	Increase benzodiazepine toxicity
Rifampin, rifabutin	Decrease benzodiazepine effect

Table continues

Table 29. ***(continued)***

Drug	Effect of Interaction
Cephalosporins	
Alcohol	Disulfiram-like reaction for those with tetrazolethiomethyl side chain: cefamandole, cefoperazone, cefotetan, cefmetazole
Aminoglycosides	Possibly increased nephrotoxicity
Ethacrynic acid	Increased nephrotoxicity
Furosemide	Increased nephrotoxicity
Clarithromycin	
Carbamazepine (Tegretol)	Increased carbamazepine levels[a]
Pimozide	Risk of ventricular arrhythmia[a]
Cisapride (Propulsid)	Risk of ventricular arrhythmias[a]
Rifabutin	Increased rifabutin levels with possible uveitis[a]
Terfenadine (Seldane)	Risk of ventricular arrhythmias[a]
Theophylline	Elevated theophylline levels
Clindamycin	
Antiperistaltic agents (Lomotil, loperamide)	Increased risk and severity of *C. difficile* colitis[a]
Clofazimine: None	
Cycloserine	
Alcohol	Increased alcohol effect or convulsions
Ethionamide	Increased CNS toxicity
Isoniazid	CNS toxicity, dizziness, drowsiness
Phenytoin	Increased phenytoin effect (toxicity)
Dapsone	
Warfarin (Coumadin)	Increased prothrombin time
ddI	Decreased levels of dapsone, give ≥2 hr apart[a]
H_2 blockers, antacids, omeprazole	Decreased absorption dapsone
Primaquine	Increased hemolysis with G-6-PD deficiency
Probenecid	Increased dapsone levels
Pyrimethamine	Increased marrow toxicity (monitor CBC)
Rifampin and rifabutin	Decreased levels of dapsone
Saquinavir	Increase dapsone levels
Trimethoprim	Increased levels of both drugs
d4T	
AZT	Possible HIV antagonism
ddC and ddI	Increased peripheral neuropathy[a]
Agents associated with peripheral neuropathy	Increased frequency and severity of peripheral neuropathy: cisplatin, ddI, ddC, dapsone, disulfiram, ethionamide, glutethimide, gold, hydralazine, iodoquinol, INH, phenytoin metronidazole (long term) vincristine

Table continues

Table 29. *(continued)*

Drug	Effect of Interaction
ddC (HIVID, zalcitabine, dideoxycytidine)	
ddI and d4T	Increased peripheral neuropathy[a]
Agents associated with peripheral neuropathy	Increased frequency and severity of peripheral neuropathy: Cisplatin, dapsone, ddI, ddC, d4T disulfiram, ethioinamide, glutethimide, gold, hydralazine, iodoquinol, INH, metronidazole, nitrofurantoin, phenytoin, vincristine[a]
Agents associated with pancreatitis	Pentamidine, ddI, rifampin
ddI (Videx, didanosine)	
Dapsone	Decreased dapsone absorption, give ≥2 hr before ddI[a]
Ganciclovir-oral	Increase ddI levels 70% (may require ddI dose reduction)
Ketoconazole, itraconazole	Decreased ketoconazole or itraconazole absorption, give ≥2 hr before ddI[a]
Indinavir	Decreased indinavir absorption, give ≥2 hrs apart
Ritonavir	Decreased ritonavir absorption, give ≥ hrs apart
Tetracycline	Decreased tetracycline absorption, give ≥2 hr before ddI[a]
Quinolones	Decreased quinolone absorption, give ≥2 hr before ddI[a]
Note: All drugs that require gastric acidity for absorption should be given ≥2 hr before or after ddI	
ddC and d4T	Increased peripheral neuropathy[a]
Agents associated with peripheral neuropathy	Increased frequency and severity of peripheral neuropathy: Cisplatin, dapsone, ddI, d4T disulfiram, ethioinamide, glutethimide, gold, hydralazine, iodoquinol, INH, metronidazole, nitrofurantoin, phenytoin, vincristine[a]
Dronabinol (Marinol)	
Alcohol	Increased CNS depression
Amphetamines, cocaine and other sympathomimetic drugs	Increased hypertension and tachycardia
Atropine, scopolamine and other anticholingergic agents	Tachycardia, drowsiness
Amitriptyline, amoxapine, other tricyclic antidepressants	Tachycardia, hypertension, drowsiness

Table continues

Table 29. *(continued)*

Drug	Effect of Interaction
Erythromycins (Inhibit cytochrome p450)	
Anticoagulants (oral)	Increased hypoprothrombinemia
Carbamazepine	Increased carbamazepine levels
Corticosteroids	Increased effect of methylprednisolone
Cyclosporine	Increased cyclosporine levels (nephrotoxicity)
Digoxin	Increased digitalis levels
Disopyramide	Increased disopyramide toxicity[a]
Ergot alkaloids	Increased ergot toxicity[a]
Phenytoin	Increased phenytoin levels
Propulsid (cisapride)	Ventricular arrhythmias[a]
Terfenadine (Seldane)	Ventricular arrhythmias[a]
Theophylline	Increased theophylline levels
Triazolam	Increased triazolam levels
Erythropoietin (EPO): None	
Ethionamide	
Cycloserine	Increased CNS levels
Isoniazid	Increased CNS levels
Fluconazole (Inhibits cytochrome p450)	
Atovaquone	Increased atovaquone levels
AZT	Increased AZT levels with fluconazole doses ≥400 mg/d
Benzodiazepines	Increased benzodiazepine levels
Clarithromycin	Increased clarithromycin levels
Warfarin (Coumadin)	Increased prothrombin time
Cyclosporine	Increased cyclosporine levels
Opiate analgesics	Increased opiate effect
Phenytoin	Increased phenytoin levels
Propulsid (cisapride)	Ventricular arrhythmias[a]
Rifabutin	Increase rifabutin levels with possible uveitis[a]
Terfenadine (Seldane)	Ventricular arrhythmias[a]
Sulfonylureas	Increased levels with hypoglycemia
Saquinavir	Increase saquinavir levels (advantage)
Fluoroquinolones (ciprofloxacin, norfloxacin, ofloxacin, lomefloxacin, enoxacin, levofloxacin, sparfloxacin)	
Antacids	Decreased fluoroquinolone absorption with Mg, Ca, or Al containing antacids or sucralfate: Give antacid >2 hr after fluoroquinolone

Table continues

Table 29. ***(continued)***

Drug	Effect of Interaction
Anticoagulants (oral)	Increased hypoprothrombinemia
Caffeine	Increased caffeine effect; primarily with ciprofloxacin and enoxacin; significance?
Cyclosporine	Possible increased nephrotoxicity
Food (dairy product)	Decrease absorption
Iron	Decreased ciprofloxacin absorption[a]
Nonsteroidal anti-inflammatory agents	Possible seizures and increased epileptogenic potential of theophylline, opiates, tricyclics, and neuroleptics
Probenecid	Increased fluoroquinolone levels
Theophylline	Increased theophylline toxicity, esp. ciprofloxacin and enoxacin (seizures, cardiac arrest, respiratory failure due to theophylline toxicity)[a]
Zinc	Decreased ciprofloxacin absorption
Fluoxetine (Prozac)	
MAO inhibitors	Risk of serotonergic syndrome—avoid initiating fluoxetine until ≥14 days after discontinuing MAO inhibitor
Astemizole	Increased astemizole levels
Warfarin (Coumadin)	Increase prothrombin time
Digitalis	Increased digitalis levels
Haloperidol	Increased haloperidol levels
Terfenadine (Seldane)	Ventricular arrhythmias[a]
Saquinavir	Increased saquinavir levels
Tricyclics	Increased tricyclic levels
Theophylline	Increased theophylline levels
Foscarnet	
Aminoglycosides	Increased renal toxicity
Amphotericin B	Increased renal toxicity
Imipenem	Increased frequency of seizures (?)
Pentamidine	Increased hypocalcemia and renal toxicity[a]
Ganciclovir	
AZT (Retrovir)	Increased leukopenia, concurrent use should be used with caution, often with G-CSF
Imipenem	Increased frequency of seizures (?)
Myelosuppressing drugs: TMP-SMX, AZT, azathrioprine, pyrimethamine, flucytosine, interferon, adriamycin, vinblastine, vincristine	Increased neutropenia
Probenecid	Increases ganciclovir levels

Table continues

Table 29. ***(continued)***

Drug	Effect of Interaction
Ganciclovir, oral	
AZT	Increased neutropenia
Food	Increased ganciclovir levels—*should be taken with meals*
Myelosuppressing drugs	See above
G-CSF and GM-CSF	
Cancer chemotherapy	Should not be given within 24 hr of chemotherapy
Indinavir (Inhibits p450 3A enzymes)	
Astemizole	Increased astemizole levels, cardiac arrhythmias[a]
Cisapride	Increased cisapride levels[a]
Didanosine (ddI)	Decreased indinavir absorption, take ≥2 hrs apart
Food	Decrease indinavir levels—take on empty stomach or with light meal without fat
Grapefruit juice	Decreased indinavir levels[a]
Midazolam (Versed)	Increased midazolam levels[a]
Rifampin and Rifabutin	Decreased indinavir levels and increased levels of rifampin or rifabutin, avoid rifampin; reduce rifabutin to half dose
Terfenadine (Seldane)	Increased terfenadine levels with cardiac arrhythmias[a]
Triazolam (Halcion)	Increased triazolam levels[a]
Antiretrovirals	
Saquinavir	Increased squinavir levels 4–7× (advantage)
Nevirapine	Indinavir levels decreased 10–30%—increase indinavir dose to 1000 mg tid
Delavirdine	Increase indinavir levels 2×—decrease indinavir dose to 600 mg tid
Nelfinavir	Nelfinavir levels increased 80×, indinavir levels increased 50%—avoid until studied
Ritonavir	No data
Nucleosides	No interaction
Interferon	
AZT	Increased marrow suppression
Barbiturates	Increased barbiturate levels
Theophylline	Increased theophylline levels
Isoniazid	
Alcohol	Increased hepatitis
	Decreased INH effect in some alcoholics
Antacids	Decreased INH levels with Al^{++} containing antacids

Table continues

Table 29. *(continued)*

Drug	Effect of Interaction
Benzodiazepines	Increased effects of benzodiazepines
Carbamazepine	Increased toxicity of both drugs[a]
Warfarin (Coumadin)	Increased hypoprothrombinemia
Cycloserine	Increased CNS toxicity, dizziness, drowsiness
Disulfiram	Psychotic episodes, ataxia[a]
Ethionamide	Increased CNS toxicity
Enflurane	Possible nephrotoxicity[a]
Food	Decreased absorption
Ketoconazole or itraconazole	Decreased azole effect[a]
Phenytoin	Increased phenytoin toxicity
Rifampin and rifabutin	Possible increased hepatic toxicity
Theophylline	Increased theophylline levels
Tyramine (foods and fluids rich in tyramine—esp. cheese, wine, some fish)	Rare patients get palpitations, sweating, urticaria, headache and/or vomiting
Itraconazole (Inhibits cytochrome p450)	
Astemizole	Increased astemizole levels
Carbamazepine (Tegretol)	Decreased itraconazole levels
Warfarin (Coumadin)	Increased hypoprothrombinemia
Cyclosporine	Increased cyclosporine levels
ddI	Decreased itraconazole levels[a]
Digoxin	Increased digoxin levels
H_2 antagonists, antacids, omeprazole	Decreased itraconazole levels does not apply to oral solution
Isoniazid	Decreased itraconazole levels[a]
Ketoconazole	Reduced ketoconazole absorption—take ≥2 hr apart
Phenobarbitol	Severe hypoglycemia
Phenytoin	Decreased itraconazole levels
Propulsid (cisapride)	Ventricular arrhythmias[a]
Rifampin or rifabutin	Decreased itraconazole levels
Terfenadine (Seldane)	Ventricular arrhythmias[a]
Ketoconazole (Inhibits cytochrome p450)	
Alcohol	Possible disulfiram-like reaction
Antacids	Decreased ketoconazole levels
Cisapride	Increased cisapride levels, ventricular arrhythmias[a]
Corticosteroids	Increased methylprednisolone levels
Warfarin (Coumadin)	Increased hypoprothrombinemia
Cyclosporine	Increased cyclosporine toxicity
ddI	Decreased ketoconazole levels—give ≥2 hours apart
H_2 antagonists, antacids, omeprazole	Decreased ketoconazole levels[a] (use sucralfate or take antacids over 2 hr before)

Table continues

Table 29. ***(continued)***

Drug	Effect of Interaction
Oral hypoglycemics	Severe hypoglycemia
Isoniazid	Decreased ketoconazole levels[a]
Indinavir	Increased indinavir levels 70%[a]
Loratadine (Claritin)	Increased levels of loratadine
Phenytoin	Altered metabolism of both drugs
Rifampin and rifabutin	Decreased activity of both drugs[a]
Saquinavir	Increased squinavir levels by 150% (advantage)
Terfenadine (Seldane)	Ventricular arrhythmias[a]
Theophylline	Increased theophylline levels
Lamivudine (3TC, Epivir)	
Trimethoprim	Increases 3TC levels 40% (implications unclear)
AZT	Resistance to 3TC promotes suceptibility to AZT—advocated combination
Megestrol: None	
Methadone	
Alcohol	Increased CNS depression
Dronabinol (Marinol)	Increased CNS depression
Marijuana	Increased CNS depression
Rifampin and rifabutin	Reduced methadone levels
Metronidazole	
Alcohol	Disulfiram-like reaction
Barbiturates	Decreased metronidazole effect with phenobarbital
Corticosteroids	Decreased metronidazole levels
Warfarin	Increased hypoprothrombinemia
Cimetidine	Possible increased metronidazole levels
Disulfiram	Organic brain syndrome[a]; stop disulfiram 2 weeks before metronidazole
Flurouracil	Transient neutropenia
Lithium	Lithium toxicity
Propulsid (cisapride)	Ventricular arrhythmias[a]
Terfenadine (Seldane)	Ventricular arrhythmias[a]
Nelfinavir (Viracept) (Inhibits cytochrome p450 3A enzymes)	
Astemizole	Ventricular arrhythmias[a]
Cisapride	Ventricular arrhythmias[a]
Ethinyl estradiol	Decreased levels; use alternative method of birth control
Midazolam	Increased midazolam levels[a]
Rifampin	Reduces nelfinavir levels substantially[a]
Rifabutin	Minimal effect on nelfinavir; rifabutin levels increased 3× —concurrent use is acceptable with rifabutin dose reduction by 50%
Triazolam	Increased levels of triazolam[a]

Table continues

Table 29. ***(continued)***

Drug	Effect of Interaction
Antiretroviral drugs	
Saquinavir	Nelfinavir levels increased 20%; saquinavir levels increased 3×—concurrent use not studied[a]
Ritonavir	Nelfinavir levels increased 2×; ritonavir levels unchanged—concurrent use not studied[a]
Indinavir	Nelfinavir levels increased 2.5×; indinavir levels increased 50%—concurrent use not studied[a]
Nucleosides	No interactions
Nystatin: None	
Paromomycin: None	
Penicillins	
Allopurinol	Increased frequency of rash with ampicillin
Contraceptives	Possible decreased contraceptive effect with ampicillin or oxacillin
Warfarin	Decreased anticoagulant effect with nafcillin and dicloxacillin
Cyclosporine	Decreased cyclosporine effect with nafcillin and increased cyclosporine toxicity with ticarcillin
Food	Decreased absorption (oral penicillin G)[a]
Lithium	Hypernatremia with ticarcillin
Methotrexate	Possible increased methotrexate toxicity
Probenecid	Increased concentrations of penicillins
Pentamidine (IV)	
Aminoglycosides	Increased nephrotoxicity[a]
Amphotericin B	Increased nephrotoxicity[a]
Capreomycin	Increased nephrotoxicity[a]
Foscarnet	Increased nephrotoxicity[a]
Pyrazinamide: None	
Pyrimethamine	
Antacids	Possible decreased pyrimethamine absorption
Dapsone	Agranulocytosis reported
Ganciclovir	Increased neutropenia
Kaolin	Possible decreased pyrimethamine absorption
Lorazepam	Hepatotoxicity
Phenothiazines	Possible chlorpromazine toxicity

Table continues

Table 29. *(continued)*

Drug	Effect of Interaction
Rifabutin (induces cytochrome p450 for increased hepatic metabolism; effect is less pronounced compared to rifampin; both drugs are also metabolized by cytochrome p450 3A so drugs that inhibit these enzymes prolong the half-life of rifabutin and rifampin); see below for drug interaction affected by this mechanism	
Clarithromycin	Increased rifabutin levels and risk of uveitis[a]
Fluconazole	Increased rifabutin levels and risk of uveitis[a]
Protease inhibitors	
Ritonavir	Increased rifabutin levels and decreased ritonavir levels[a]
Indinavir	Increased rifabutin levels—reduce rifabutin dose 50%
Saquinavir	Increased rifabutin levels, reduced saquinavir levels[a]
Rifampin (induces cytochrome p450 hepatic enzymes; also metabolized by cytochrome p450 enzymes)	
Aminosalicyclic acid (PAS)	Decreased effectiveness of rifampin; give in separate doses ×8–12 hr
Atovaquone	Decreased atovaquone levels
Barbiturates	Decreased barbiturate levels
Benzodiazepines	Possible decreased benzodiazepine levels
β-Adrenergic blockers	Decreased β blocker levels
Chloramphenicol	Decreased chloramphenicol levels[a]
Clofazimine	Reduced rifampin levels
Clofibrate	Decreased clofibrate levels
Contraceptives	Decreased contraceptive effect[a]
Corticosteroids	Decreased corticosteroid levels[a]
Warfarin	Decreased hypoprothrombinemia
Cyclosporine	Decreased cyclosporine levels[a]
Dapsone	Decreased dapsone levels
Digitalis	Decreased digitalis levels
Disopyramide	Decreased disopyramide levels[a]
Doxycycline	Decreased doxycycline levels
Haloperidol	Decreased haloperidol levels
Hypoglycemics	Decreased hypoglycemic effect
Indinavir	Reduced indinavir levels and increased rifampin levels[a]
Isoniazid	Increased hepatoxicity
Ketoconazole	Decreased levels of ketoconazole and rifampin[a]

Table continues

Table 29. *(continued)*

Drug	Effect of Interaction
Methadone	Methadone withdrawal symptoms[a]
Mexiletine	Decreased antiarrhythnmic effect
Phenytoin	Decreased phenytoin levels
Progestins	Decreased norethindrone levels
Quinidine	Decreased quinidine levels
Ritonavir	Reduced ritonavir levels and increased rifampin levels[a]
Saquinavir	Decrease saquinavir levels and increased rifampin levels[a]
Theophylline	Decreased theophylline levels
Trimethoprim	Decreased trimethoprim levels
Trimetrexate	Decreased trimetrexate levels
Verapamil	Decreased verapamil levels
Ritonavir (Profound inhibition of p450 cytochromes including 3A and 2D6; this is also the major mechanism of ritonavir metabolism). Drugs that should *not* be co-administered: Meperidine (Demerol), piroxicam (Feldene), Darvon, amiodarone, encainide, flecainide, propafenone, quinidine, rifabutin, bepridil (Vascor), astemizole, terfenadine (Seldane), cisapride (Propulsid), bupropion (Wellbutrin), clozapine, alprazolam (Xanax), clorazepate (Tranxene), diazepam (Valium), flurazepam (Dalmane), estazolam, midazolam (Versed), triazolam (Halcion) zolpidem (Ambien), pimozide and ergot alkaloids	
Carbamazepine	Decreased ritonavir levels
Clarithromycin	Increase clarithromycin levels
Warfarin	Increased anticoagulant effect
Delavirdine	No significant interaction—standard doses of each
Desipramine	Increased desipramine levels—reduce dose of desipramine
Dexamethasone	Decreased ritonavir levels and decreased corticosteroid level
Didanosine	Reduced ritonavir absorption; take ≥2 hrs apart
Erythromycin	Increased erythromycin levels
Fentanyl	Increased fentanyl levels
Food	Modest increase in ritonavir levels—take with meals
Ketoconazole	Increased ketoconazole levels—dose adjustment only with renal failure
Methadone	Possible increase methadone levels
Nelfinavir	Nelfinavir levels increase 2×; no change in ritonavir levels
Nevirapine	No significant interaction—standard doses of each

Table continues

Table 29. *(continued)*

Drug	Effect of Interaction
Oral contraceptives	Reduced estradiol levels: use alternative method of contraception
Oxycodone	Increased oxycodone levels
Phenobarbitol	Decreased ritonavir levels
Phenytoin	Decreased ritonavir levels
Rifampin	Decreased ritonavir levels
Saquinavir	Increase in saquinavir levels >20× (advantage); regimen for concurrent use if saquinavir 400 mg bid and ritonavir 400–600 mg bid
Theophylline	Reduced theophylline levels—increase dose of theophylline
Tricyclic antidepressants	Moderate increase tricyclic level
Saquinavir (Poor bioavailability due to reduced absorption and hepatic metabolism by cytochrome p450. Drugs that inhibit p450 promote bioavailability; those that induce p450 should be avoided); a soft gel capsule formulation with increased bioavailability is expected in 1997)	
Astemizole	Increase levels both drugs[a]
Carbamazepine	Decreased saquinavir levels
Clindamycin	Increased clindamycin levels
Cisapride	Increased cisapride levels[a]
Dapsone	Increased dapsone levels
Delavirdine	Increased saquinavir levels 5× (advantage)
Dexamethasone	Decrease saquinavir levels
Food	Fat meal improves bioavailability
Fluconazole	Increase saquinavir levels
Grapefruit juice	Increases saquinavir levels
Indinavir	Increase saquinavir 4–7×, no effect on indinavir levels
Ketoconazole	Increase saquinavir levels 150% (advantage)
Nevirapine	Decrease saquinavir levels[a]
Nelfinavir	Nelfinavir levels increase 20%; saquinavir levels increase 3×—standard doses
Phenobarbital	Decreased saquinavir levels
Phenytoin	Decreased saquinavir levels
Rifabutin	Decreased saquinavir levels by 40%; consider alternative
Rifampin	Decreased saquinavir levels by 80%[a]
Ritonavir	Increased levels of both drugs; regimen for concurrent use is saquinavir 400 mg bid plus ritonavir 400–600 mg bid

Table continues

Table 29. ***(continued)***

Drug	Effect of Interaction
Terfenadine (Seldane)	Increased terfenadine levels with possible ventricular arrhythmias[a]
Serostim (growth hormone)—drug interactions have not been studied	
Sulfonamides	
Barbiturates	Increased thiopental levels
Warfarin	Increased hypoprothrombinemia
Cyclosporine	Decreased cyclosporine levels with sulfamethazine
Digoxin	Decreased digoxin levels with sulfasalazine
Hypoglycemic, oral	Increased hypoglycemic effect of sulfonylurea
Methotrexate	Increased methotrexate levels
Monoamine oxidase inhibitors	Increased phenelzine levels with sulfisoxazole
Phenytoin	Increased phenytoin levels except with sulfisoxazole
Tetracycline	
Alcohol	Decreased doxycycline levels in alcoholics
Antacids	Decreased tetracycline levels with antacids containing Ca^{++}, Al^{++}, Mg^{++}, and $NaHCO_3$
Antidepressants, tricyclic	Localized hemosiderosis with amitriptyline and minocycline
Anti-diarrhea agents	Agents containing kaolin and pectin or bismuth subsalicylate, decreased tetracycline levels
Barbiturates	Decreased doxycycline levels[a]
Bismuth subsalicylate (Pepto-Bismol)	Decreased tetracycline levels[a]
Carbamazepine (Tegreotol)	Decreased doxycycline levels[a]
Contraceptives, oral	Decreased contraceptive effect (? significance)
Warfarin	Increased hypoprothrombinemia
Digoxin	Increased digoxin levels (10% of population)
Iron, oral	Decreased tetracycline levels and decreased iron effect; give 3 hr before
Laxatives	Agents containing Mg^{++} decrease tetracycline levels
Lithium	Possible increased lithium toxicity (single case)
Methotrexate	Increased methotrexate levels
Methoxyflurane anesthesia (Penthrane)	Possibly lethal nephrotoxicity[a]

Table continues

Table 29. *(continued)*

Drug	Effect of Interaction
Milk	Decreased absorption of tetracycline[a] Does *not* apply to doxycycline or minocycline
Molindone	Decreased tetracycline levels
Phenformin	Decreased doxycycline levels[a]
Phenytoin	Decreased doxycycline levels
Rifampin and rifabutin	Possible decreased doxycycline levels
Theophylline	Increased theophylline levels
Zinc	Decreased tetracycline levels[a]
Trimethoprim	
Amantadine	Increased levels of both drugs
Azathioprine	Leukopenia
Cyclosporine	Increased nephrotoxicity[a]
Dapsone	Increased levels of both drugs; increased methemoglobinemia
Digoxin	Possible increased digitalis levels
Phenytoin	Increased phenytoin levels
Rifampin	Decreased trimethoprim levels
Thiazide diuretics	Possible increased hyponatremia with concomitant use of amiloride with thiazide diuretics
Trimethoprim-sulfamethoxazole	
Warfarin	Increased hypoprothrombinemia
Ganciclovir	Increased neutropenia
Mercaptopurine	Decreased mercaptopurine levels
Methotrexate	Megaloblastic anemia[a]
Phenytoin	Increased phenytoin levels[a]
Procainamide	Increased procainamide
Trimetrexate	
Acetaminophen	Increased trimetrexate levels
AZT	Increased bone marrow suppression
Cimetidine	Increased trimetrexate levels
Erythromycin	Increased trimetrexate levels
Fluconazole	Increased trimetrexate levels
Ketoconazole	Increased trimetrexate levels
Rifampin, rifabutin	Decreased trimetrexate levels
Vancomycin	
Aminoglycosides	Increased nephrotoxicity and possible increased ototoxicity[a]
Amphotericin B	Increased nephrotoxicity
Cisplatin	Increased nephrotoxicity
Digoxin	Decreased digoxin levels

Adapated from the Medical Letter Handbook of Adverse Drug Interactions—1991: 6–282, 1991; package inserts from suppliers; AMA Drug Evaluations and Drug Information 94. Am Soc Hosp Pharmacist, Bethesda, MD, 1996; CID 1996;23:685.
[a] Concurrent use should be avoided if possible.

** Does not apply to Sporanox Oral Solution

Table 30. Drug Information, Treatment INDs, and Financial Assistance Programs

Drug	Program	Contact
Acyclovir (Zovirax)	Cap Program: Individual use >552 g[a]	800-722-9294
	Patient assistance	800-722-9294
Albendazole	Microsporidosis—available from Smith Kline	800-877-7074
Atovaquone (Mepron)	Patient assistance[b]	800-722-9294
Azithromycin (Zithromax)	Treatment IND for cryptosporidiosis toxoplasmosis and disseminated MAC	215-972-0420
	Patient assistance[b]	800-646-4455
AZT (Retrovir)	Patient assistance	800-722-9294
Cidofovir (HPMPC) (Vistide)	Patient assistance	800-445-3235
Ciprofloxacin (Cipro)	Patient assistance	800-998-9180
Clarithromycin (Biaxin)	Patient assistance	800-688-9118
D4T (Stavudine) (Zerit)	Patient assistance[b]	800-272-4878
Doxil (Liposomal doxorubicin)	Ordering	800-458-4390
	Patient assistance—KS refractory to standard treatment	800-375-1658
ddI (Videx) (didanosine)	Patient assistance[b]	800-272-4878
ddC (HIVID) (Zalcitabine)	Patient assistance[b]	800-282-7780
EPO (Procrit)	Patient assistance	800-553-3851
EPO (Epogen)	Patient assistance	800-272-9376
Fluconazole (Diflucan)	Patient assistance[b]	800-869-9979 or 800-646-4455
Foscarnet (Foscavir)	Patient assistance	800-488-3247
Ganciclovir (IV and oral)	Patient assistance	800-285-4484
Ganciclovir intraocular Implant	Patient assistance	800-843-1137
G-CSF (Neupogen)	Reimbursement assistance and Patient assistance[b]	800-272-9376
GM-CSF (Leukine)	Patient assistance[b]	800-321-4669
Indinavir	Patient assistance	800-850-3430
	Product information	800-497-8383
Interferon	Patient assistance	800-443-6676
(Roferon)	Cap Program: 983 million units[a]	800-443-6676
(Intron)	Product information and Patient assistance[b]	800-521-7157
Itraconazole (Sporonox)	Patient assistance[b]	800-544-2987
Ketoconazole (Nizoral)	Patient assistance[b]	800-544-2987
Lamivudine (3TC)	Patient assistance[b]	800-722-9294
Marinol (Dronabinol)	Patient assistance[b]	800-274-8651
Megace (Megestrol)	Patient assistance[b]	800-426-7644
Nevirapine	Patient assistance[b]	800-274-8651

Table continues

Table 30. *(continued)*

Drug	Program	Contact
Octreotide (Sandostatin)	Patient assistance[b]	800-447-6677
Pentamidine	Patient assistance—aerosolized pentamidine[b]	708-317-8604
	Reimbursement hotline	800-366-6323
Retrovir (AZT)	Patient assistance[b]	800-722-9294
Rifabutin	Patient assistance[b]	800-366-5570
Ritonavir	Patient assistance[b]	800-659-9050
Saquinavir (Invirase)	Reimbursement hotline and Patient assistance	800-282-7780
Serostim (growth hormone)	Patient assistance and annual $36,000 cap	800-714-2437
Streptomycin	Free supply (Pfizer)	800-254-4445
Sulfadiazine	(Now available from Eon Labs)	718-276-8600
3TC (Lamivudine)	Patient assistance	800-722-9294
	Patient assistance	800-513-3028
	Insurance/claims assistance	800-513-3028
Thalidomide	Treatment IND	301-827-2335
	Apthous ulcers: FDA approval Supplier: Andrulis Pharm Inc	301-419-2400
	Wasting— Supplier: Celgene	800-801-8328
Trimetrexate	Patient assistance Reimbursement information	800-887-2467

[a] Cap program: Free drug will be provided when cumulative designated dose or wholesale cost is used in <1 yr; the free supply will be provided until the 1-yr anniversary date.
[b] Usual requirements are lack of prescription drug insurance (including state plans and Ryan White funds) usually accompanied with income/asset criteria.

7—Major Complications of HIV Infection

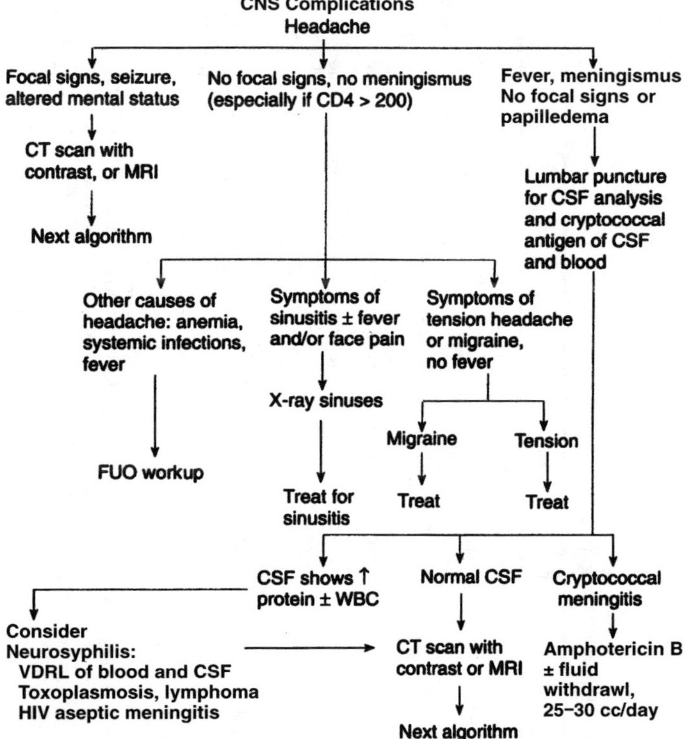

Figure 2. Headache. *CT,* computerized tomography; *MRI,* magnetic resonance imaging; *CSF,* cerebrospinal fluid; *FUO,* fever of unknown origin; *WBC,* white blood cell count; *VDRL,* venereal disease research laboratory; *5FC,* 5-flucytosine.

Table 31. CNS Infection: Differential Diagnosis

Agent	Course	Frequency Setting	Typical Findings	Diagnosis
Toxoplasmosis	Acute	Common: 3–10% of all AIDS patients; 20–35% of AIDS patients with CD4 <100, plus positive serology without prophylaxis	Mental status: reduced; temp: fever; scan: ring-enhanced lesions with mass effect and usually multiple lesions widely distributed; CSF: increased protein and 0–40 monos; nl 25%	Typical clinical and scan findings: response to empiric treatment with clinical improvement in ≤1 wk or scan improvement in 2 wks; IgG serology positive in 85–95%; toxo PCR in CSF
Lymphoma	Typically subacute	3% of all AIDS patients CD4 <100	Mental status: variable; temp: afebrile; scan: solid-enhanced lesions with mass effect; location: periventricular, multiple in 60% CSF: increased protein and 0–100 monos; nl 40%	Typical clinical and scan findings ± failure to respond to empiric treatment of toxoplasmosis; PCR for EBV in CSF
PML	Subacute	1–3% of all AIDS patients, CD4 <100	Mental status: Alert; temp: afebrile; scan: punctate, nonenhanced discrete multifocal lesions without mass effect; location: subcortical white matter; CSF: normal	Typical clinical and scan findings; stereotactic biopsy-antibody to SV40; characteristic inclusions in oligodendrocytes.
Cryptococcal	Acute, subacute, or chronic	Common: 8–12% of all AIDS patients; CD4 <100 median-20	Mental status: alert; temp: fever; scan: no focal lesions; location: basal ganglia; CSF: increase protein, 0–100 monos, decreased glucose, nl in 20%	CSF: cryptococcal antigen and positive culture: blood: crypt antigen positive in >90% with meningitis

AIDS dementia complex (ADC)	Subacute or chronic	20–30% of all AIDS patients: CD4 < 100	Mental status: alert; temp` afebrile; scan: atrophy and ill-defined changes of deep white matter; location: deep white matter; CSF: increased protein and 5–10 monos, Beta 2 microglobulin >3 mg/L; nl 40%	Neuropsychiatric tests show subcortical dementia combined with typical scan; mini-mental is insensitive
CMV encephalitis	Acute	1–2% of all AIDS patients; CD4 <50	Mental status: delirious; temp: afebrile; hyponatremia; —due to CMV adrenalitis; scan: periventricular infection; CSF: increased protein, decreased glucose, 10–1000 monos	CSF: cultures negative PCR usually positive; typical clinic setting and scan: empiric anti-CMV therapy
Neurosyphilis	Asymptomatic Meningeal Tabes dorsalis General paresis Meningovascular Ocular	0.5%; any stage	Variable with stage CSF: increased protein, 5–100 monos ±VDRL	Blood VDRL and FTA-ABS pos typical CSF changes CSF VDRL + in 65% specificity—100%; CSF: Pos VDRL is diagnostic; one third have false-neg VDRL
Tuberculosis	Chronic	0.5–1%	Mental status: reduced; temp: fever; scan intracerebral enhancing lesions in 50–70%; CSF: increased protein, 5–2000 monos; decreased glucose, nl 5–10%	Chest x-ray; Culture pos from any site; CSF cult pos in 20%; PPD variable

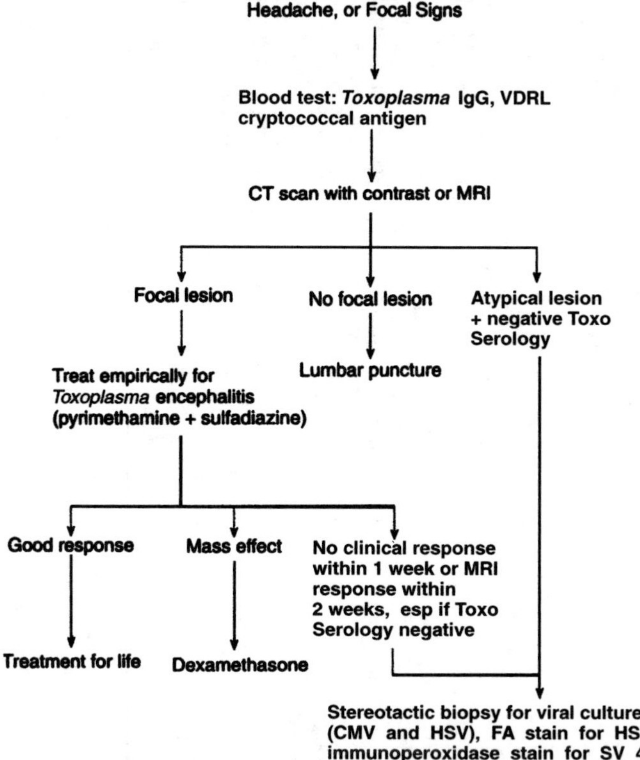

Figure 3. CNS evaluation. *CT*, computerized tomography; *MRI*, magnetic resonance imaging; *FA*, fluorescent antibody; *PML*, polymorphonuclear leukocyte.

Pulmonary Complications

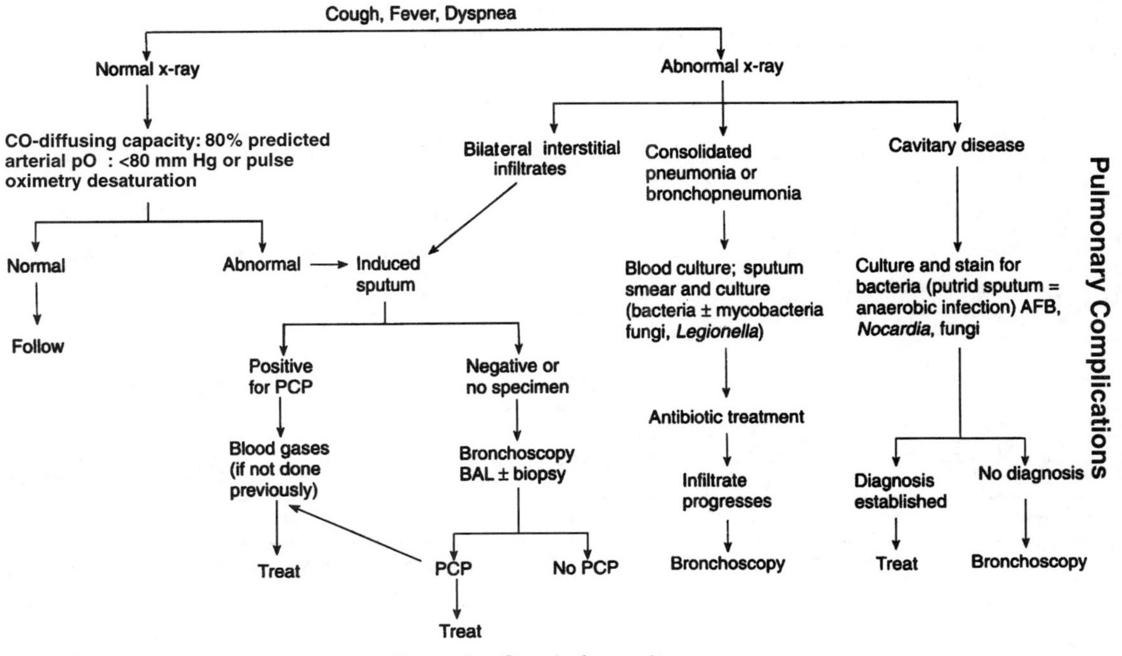

Figure 4. Cough, fever, dyspnea.

Table 32. Pulmonary Infection: Differential Diagnosis

Agent	Course[a]	Frequency Setting	Typical Findings	Diagnosis[b]
Bacteria				
S. pneumoniae	Acute	Common, all stages HIV infection	Lobar or bronchopneumonia ± pleural effusion	Sputum GS, Quellung, culture, blood culture
H. influenzae	Acute	Moderately common; all stages HIV infection	Bronchopneumonia	Sputum GS and culturre
Gram-neg bacilli	Acute	Uncommon, except with nosocomial infection, neutropenia, cavity, chronic antibiotic exposure, or late stage disease (esp *P. aeruginosa*)	Lobar or bronchopneumonia, cavity	Sputum GS and culture
Legionella[c]	Acute	Unusual except in epidemic and endemic areas	Bronchopneumonia multiple noncontiguous segments	Sputum DFA stain and/or culture; urinary antigen (*L. pneumophila*, type 1)
S. aureus	Acute	Uncommon except with influenza or tricuspid valve endocarditis with septic emboli	Bronchopneumonia or multiple nodules ± cavitation	Blood cultures (endocarditis), sputum GS and culture
Nocardia[c]	Chronic or asymptomatic	Uncommon; late stage HIV	Nodule or cavity	Sputum or FOB; GS, modified AFB stain and culture
Mycobacteria Tuberculosis (MTB)[c]	Chronic, subacute, or asymptomatic	Moderate ↑ IVDA urban areas; all stages—mean CD4 is 200–300/mm^3; extrapulmonary TB common	Variable: focal infiltrates, reticular, cavity disease, hilar adenopathy, lower and middle lobe involvement common, pleural effusion	Sputum AFB stain and culture; induced sputum or bronchoscopy

M. avium	Chronic	Moderate (see diagnosis); CD4 <50	Variable	Recovery in sputum or FOB: must distinguish from MTB (DNA or radiometric culture technique); MA may colonize airways without causing pulmonary disease
M. kansasii	Chronic or asymptomatic	Uncommon: late-stage HIV CD4 < 50	Cavity disease, nodule, cyst, infiltrate	Recovery in sputum or FOB
Fungi				
Cryptococcus	Chronic, subacute, or asymptomatic	Moderately common: advanced HIV infection; with median CD4 of 50; 80% have cryptococcal meningitis	Nodule, cavity, diffuse, or nodular infiltrates	Sputum or FOB stain and culture; serum cryptococcal antigen; LP indicated
Histoplasma capsulatum[c]	Chronic or subacute	Uncommon outside endemic area; usually advanced HIV infection with disseminated histoplasmosis—median CD4 is 50	Diffuse or nodular infiltrates, nodule, focal infiltrate, cavity, hilar adenopathy	Sputum or FOB stain and culture; serum and urine antigen assay, serology; highest yield with culture: marrow
Coccidioides immitis[c]	Chronic or subacute	Uncommon outside endemic area; median CD4-50 advanced HIV infection	Diffuse or nodular infiltrates, focal infiltrate, cavity, hilar adenopathy	Sputum or FOB stain and culture, serology

Table 32. *(continued)*

Agent	Course[a]	Frequency Setting	Typical Findings	Diagnosis[b]
Candida	Chronic or subacute	Common isolate, rare cause of pulmonary disease; median CD4 50	Bronchitis; rare cause of pulmonary infiltrate	Recovery in sputum or FOB specimen is meaningless; should have histological evidence of invasion on biopsy
Aspergillus	Acute or subacute	Up to 4% of patients with advanced HIV infection; corticosteroids and neutropenia (ANC <500/mm^3)	Focal infiltrate, cavity often pleural-based	Sputum stain and culture: false-positive and false-negative cultures common; most reliable are positive stain in typical setting or biopsy evidence of tissue invasion
Virus				
CMV	Subacute or chronic	Common isolate, rare cause of pulmonary disease; advanced HIV infection with median CD4 <20	Interstitial infiltrates	Yield of CMV by cytopath or culture with FOB is 20–50%; diagnosis of CMV pneumonitis requires CMV by biopsy, or CMV plus progressive disease *and* no alternative pathogen
Influenza[c]	Acute	Influenza is common; influenza pneumonia is rare; any stage of HIV infection; frequency and course similar to patients without HIV infection	URI, pharyngitis, bronchitis—most common. Bronchopneumonia, terstitial infiltrates are rare except with bacterial superinfection	Culture of throat washing. FA stain of sputum serology, epidemiology in community and typical symptoms

HSV, VZV, RSV, paraflu	Acute	Rare causes of pneumonia	Diffuse or nodular pneumonia, bronchopneumonia	Culture of sputum or FOB commonly yields HSV as a contaminant from upper airways
Parasite				
Pneumocystis[c]	Subacute or chronic	Very common in late stages of HIV infection (CD4 <200; median CD4 130 without prophylaxis, 30 with prophylaxis	Interstitial infiltrates; negative x-ray in 10–30%; atypical findings; upper lobe infiltrates, focal infiltrates especially in patients receiving aerosolized pentamidine; also has ↑ LDH (90%), ↓ pO_2 (95%), ↓ pulse oximitry ↓ diffusing capacity	Cytopath of induced sputum or FOB; yield with induced sputum 40–80% (average 60%) and depends on quality assurance; yield with FOB BAL: >95%
Miscellaneous				
Kaposi's sarcoma	Chronic or asymptomatic	Moderately common in patients with cutaneous KS	Interstitial, alveolar, or nodular infiltrates; hilar adenopathy pleural effusions; gallium scan usually negative	FOB: endobronchial lesion often seen; yield with FOB biopsy of parenchymal lesion is only 10–30%
Lymphoma	Chronic or asymptomatic	Uncommon, but may be presenting site	Interstitial, alveolar, or nodular infiltrates; cavity, hilar adenopathy, pleural effusions	FOB: yield very poor; open lung biopsy usually required
Lymphocytic interstitial pneumonia (LIP)	Chronic or subacute	Uncommon in adults	Diffuse reticular infiltrates, focal infiltrate	FOB: yield with biopsy is 30–50%; open lung biopsy often required

[a] Course: Acute—symptoms evolve over days; subacute—symptoms evolve over 2–6 weeks; chronic—symptoms evolve over >4 weeks.
[b] Diagnosis: *Expectorated sputum* for bacterial culture should have cytological screening to show predominance of PMN; Gram stain (GS) and Quellung (if GS suggest *S. pneumoniae*). *Induced sputum* is usually reserved for patients with nonproductive cough and suspected PCP or *M. tuberculosis, Fiberoptic bronchoscopy* (FOB) assumes bronchoveolar lavage spcimen (BAL) ± touch preps, bronchial washings, bronchial brush, or transbronchial biopsy; the usual spcimen for PCP is BAL. Detection of *fungi* includes stains (KOH and/or Gomori methenamine silver stain) and culture (Sabouraud's media); *Candida* sp. grow on conventional bacteria media. Detection of *viruses* includes cytopathology for inclusions (herpes viruses-CMV, HSV, VZV); FA for HSV and influenza; cultures are for herpes viruses and with special request—influenza virus.
[c] Detection of these organisms in respiratory secretions is essentially diagnostic of disease; other organisms may be contaminants, colonizing mucosal surfaces or commensals.

Table 33. Oral Lesions: Differential Diagnosis

Condition	Clinical Features	Diagnosis
Candidiasis (Thrush)	White plaques on inflammed base; CD4 count <300 ± antibiotics	Usually a clinical dx; KOH or gram stain shows yeast and pseudomycelia
Oral hairy leukoplakia (OHL)	White hairlike projections usually on lateral surface of tongue; CD4 count <300	Usually a clinical dx and often mistaken for thrush. Bx shows hairlike projections with EBV by FA stain
Herpes simplex	Small painful vesicles on inflammed base, esp palate or gingiva; any CD4 count, but chronic and severe with <100	Usually a clinical diagnosis in patient with hx of "cold sores"\Smear will show multinucleate giant cells with HSV by FA stain and culture
Aphthous ulcers	Crops of painful ulcers on mucosal surface; any CD4 count	Negative evaluation for HSV, CMV, VZV
Kaposi's sarcoma	Purple or black nodules usually on palate or gingiva; CD4 count <300	Clinical appearance. Biopsy may confirm dx

Table 34. Dysphagia/Odynophagia: Differential Diagnosis

Condition	Clinical Features	Diagnosis
Candida esophagitis	Accounts for 50–70%. Usually has: Thrush, diffuse esophageal pain, afebrile, CD4 count <100	Usually a presumed dx with odynophagia + thrush Endoscopy—white plaques, brushing or hx shows yeast
CMV	Accounts for 10–20%. Pain is focal and severe, fever is common, CD4 count <100	Bx required for treatment Endoscopy shows one or multiple ulcers, bx shows CMV inclusions; culture not recommended
Herpes simplex (HSV)	Accounts for 2–5%. Usually has oral ulcers, focal pain, fever uncommon, CD4 count <100	Endoscopy shows small confluent ulcers, bx show HSV inclusions pos FA stain and culture
Idiopathic (Aphthous ulcers)	Accounts for 10–20%. Focal pain, afebrile, CD4 count variable	Negative evaluation for pathogens Endoscopy—appears like CMV

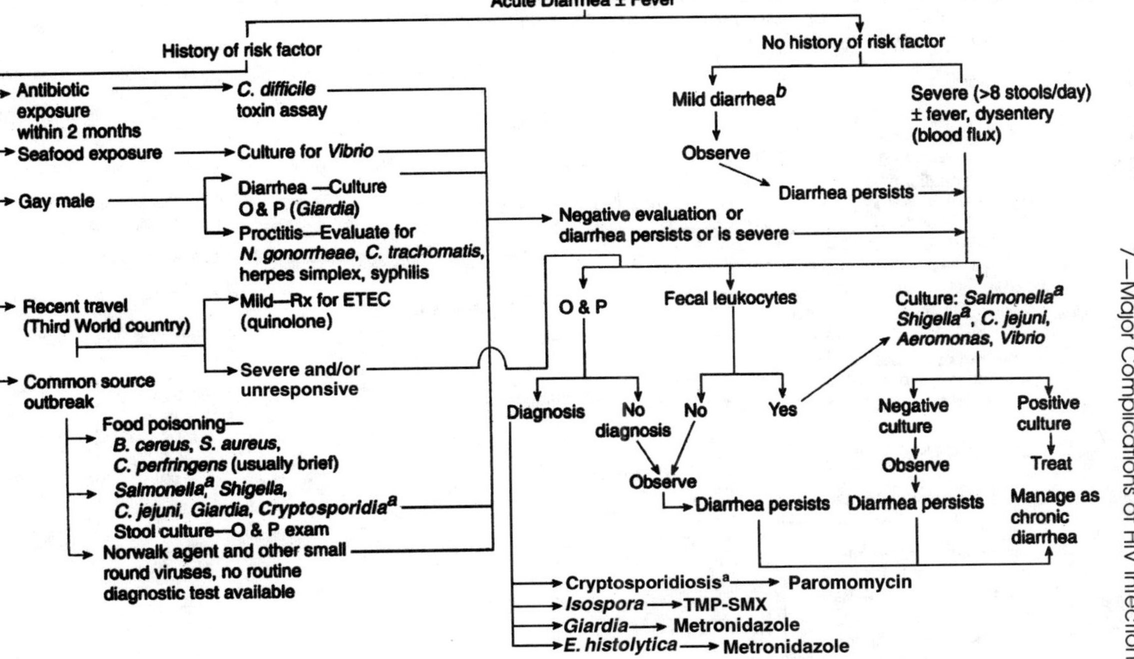

Figure 5. Acute diarrhea with or without fever.

[a] Pathogens considered more frequent and/or severe in patients with advanced HIV infection.

[b] Most diarrhea is due to medications, anxiety, irritable bowel syndrome, or untreatable viral agents (Norwalk agent, other small round viruses, etc.); factors that increase the likelihood of a treatable pathogen are severity of diarrhea, presence of fever, and fecal leukocytes and/or blood.

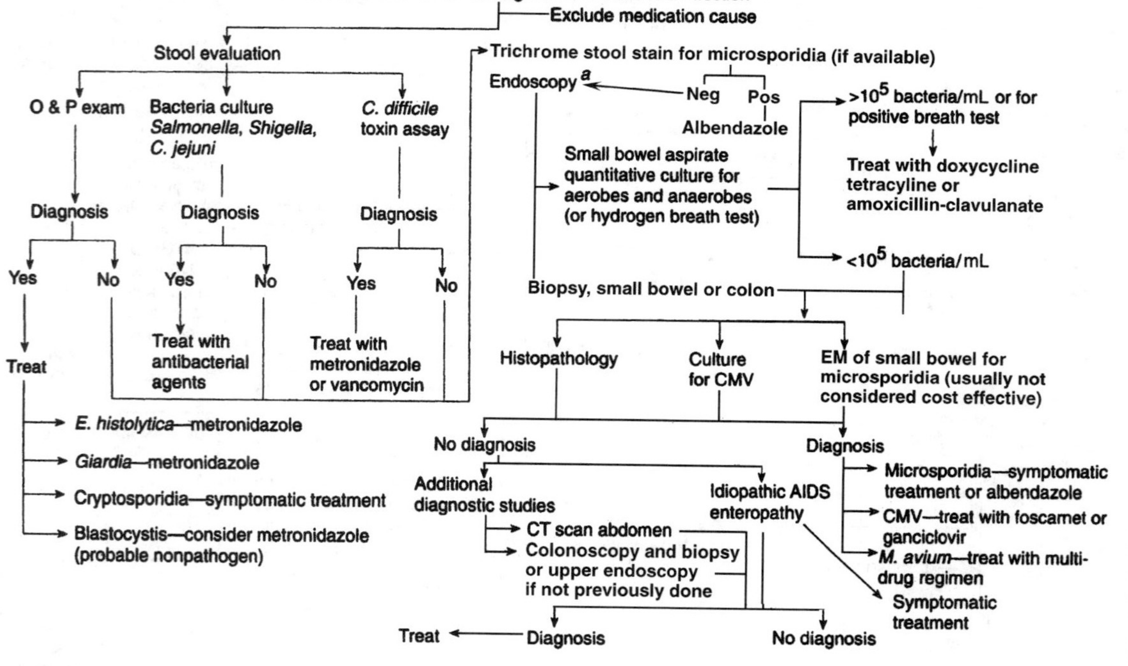

Figure 6. Chronic diarrhea with or without wasting with advanced HIV infection.

[a] Lower endoscopy is appropriate as initial endoscopy procedure if there is evidence of colonic disease by symptoms (cramps, dysentery, tenesmus), fecal white blood cells, fecal blood, or computerized tomography (CT) scan. Upper endoscopy is preferred if there is large volume diarrhea without fever or cramps and negative fecal WBC exam.

Table 35. Diarrhea: Differential Diagnosis

Agent	Course[a]	Frequency/Setting	Typical Findings	Diagnosis[b]
Bacteria				
Salmonella	Acute or subacute	5–15% of acute diarrheas; any stage of HIV	Enteric fever or gastroenteritis	Blood and stool culture; fecal WBC variable
Shigella	Acute	1–3% of acute diarrheas; any CD4 count	Dysentery (blood and mucus); fever common; colitis	Stool culture; fecal WBC usually present
C. jejuni	Acute	4–8% of acute diarrheas; any CD4 cell count	Stools watery or dysenteric; fever variable; colitis	Stool culture; fecal WBC often present
C. difficile	Acute or chronic	10–15% of acute diarrheas; virtually always with antibiotic exposure, esp. clindamycin, ampicillin or cephalosporins	Stools watery; fever and leukocytosis common; colitis	*C. difficile* toxin assay; fecal WBC variable
Small bowel overgrowth	Chronic	Frequency unknown	Stools watery; no fever malabsorption	Small bowel aspirate for quantitative culture and/or hydrogen breath test; fecal WBC negative
Mycobacteria				
M. avium	Chronic	10–20% of chronic diarrheas; CD4 <50	Watery diarrhea; enteritis	Most patients have MAC bacteremia Small bowel biopsy with AFB strain ± culture; fever, abdominal pain, Hepatomegaly
Parasites				
Cryptosporidia	Acute or chronic	20–30% of chronic diarrheas CD4 <200	Stools watery, up to 20 Liters/day usually afrebrile, enteritis	Stool AFB or DFA stain; shows typical oocytes; fecal WBC negative
Isospora	Chronic	1–2% of chronic diarrheas; CD4 <100	Stools watery, fever uncommon; enteritis	Stool AFB smear, fecal WBC negative

Table 35. ***(continued)***

Agent	Course[a]	Frequency/Setting	Typical Findings	Diagnosis[b]
Microsporidia	Chronic	15–20% of chronic diarrheas; CD4<50	Stools watery, fever uncommon, enteritis	Trichrome stain of stool to detect microsporidia "Gold standard" is EM of small bowel bx (or Giemsa stain)
Giardia	Chronic	1–2% of chronic diarrheas; more common in gay men and travelers; any CD4 count	Watery diarrhea ± malabsorption; no fever; symptoms include bloating, flatulence; enteritis	Stool O & P exam; Giardia antigen assay
E. histolytica	Chronic or subacute	1–2% of chronic diarrheas more common in gay men and travelers; any CD4 count	Asymptomatic carriage common, esp. in gay men; symptoms include bloody stools and fever; colitis	Stool O & P exam; stool shows RBCs; ability of techs to find trophs highly variable—suggest three stool specimens, endoscopy with scraping or biopsy; serology—IFA titer ↑
Cyclospora cayetanensis	Chronic	<1% of chronic diarrheas	Watery diarrhea	AFB on stool shows circular organisms larger than cryptosporidia
Viruses				
CMV	Chronic or subacute	10–40% of chronic diarrheas; CD4 count <50	Enteritis or colitis; represents disseminated CMV; fever, pain, may cause colonic perforation, acute bleed	Intestinal biopsy to show CMV inclusions ± culture; CMV sometimes seen in absence of inflammation or symptoms

Enteric viruses	Acute or chronic	15–30% of acute diarrheas; any CD4 count	Enteritis; watery diarrhea	Major agents cannot be detected by clinical labs—astrovirus, adenoviruses, caliciviruses, picobirnavirus
Idiopathic	Chronic	20–30% of chronic diarrheas	Watery diarrhea, small intestinal biopsy shows ↓ villus; crypt ratio witout ↑ intraepithelial lymphocytes	Diagnosis based on typical histological changes and negative studies for microbial cause

[a] Course: Chronic indicates diarrhea for most days during ≥1 month.

[b] Diagnosis: 1) Stool culture in most labs includes selective media for *Shigella, Salmonella,* and *C. jejuni* ± E. coli 0157, *Aeromonas, Pleisomonas, Yersina,* and *Vibrios.* 2) The preferred test for *C. difficile* is the EIA or tissue culture assay. 3) O & P exam should be done in fresh stool or stool fixed with polyvinyl alcohol. 4) Modified AFB stain detects *Cryptosporidia, Isospora, Cyclospora,* and *M. avium.* 5) Fecal WBC exam distinguishes "inflammatory" and "secretory" diarrheas: a positive result specifically suggests CMV *Salmonella, Shigella, C. jejuni, C. difficile, Yersina, Aeromonas, Vibrio parahemolyticus.* 6) Serology is useful primrily for *E. histolytica* using IFA, which is increased in 85% with amebic colitis. Endoscopy includes protoscopy, sigmoidoscopy, colonoscopy, and small bowel endoscopy; these are in ascending order of cost and diagnostic utility for unselected AIDS patients and diarrhea. Proctoscopy is preferred for patients with proctitis (usually due to STDs, including *N. gonorrhoeae, Chlamydia trachomatis,* herpes simplex, and syphilis); small bowel endoscopy with duodenal biopsy has highest yield in patients with "noninflammatory" chronic diarrhea in late stages of HIV infections; and colonoscopy or sigmoidoscopy is preferred in patients with evidence of colitis (i.e., pain, fever, tenesmus, bloody stools, and/or fecal leukocytes).

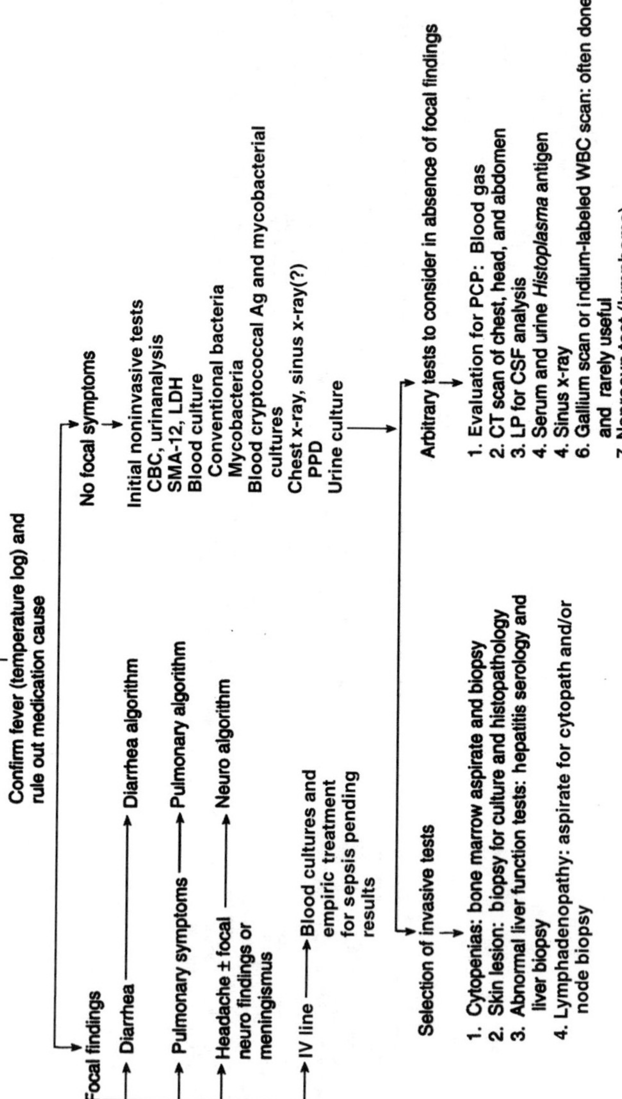

Figure 7. Fever of unknown origin (*FUO*).

Table 36. Dermatologic Complications: Differential Diagnosis

Condition	Presentation	Diagnosis
Adverse drug reaction	Red, papular, pruritic rash most common. Less common: urticaria, erythema multiforme, photosensitivity Any CD4 count	Response to drug holiday usually adequate unless severe or unresponsive Association with drugs, esp TMP-SMX, dapsone, nevaripine, delavirdine
Bacillary angiomatosis	Papules or nodules. Resembles KS CD4 variable, usually <200	Bx: Warthin—Starry stain shows *B. henseiae* Responds to erythromycin
Cryptococcosis	Noduler, ulcerative or vesicular lesions may resemble HSV, VZV or molluscum CD4 <100	BX—methenamine stain shows yeast
Eosinophilic folliculitis	Pruritic papules and pustules; CD4 <250	Bx: Eosinophilic infiltrate in follicular epithelium
Herpes simplex	Vesicles with erythematous base—oral, genital, perirectal or general cutaneous Chronicity and severity inversely related to CD4 count	Tzanck prep showing multinucleate giant cells; FA stain and/or culture for HSV ± sensitivity tests in refractory cases Biopsy
Herpes zoster	Vesicles on erythematous base in dermatomal distribution. Complications are pain, including post herpetic neuralgia, disseminated disease, blindness; any CD4 count	Tzank prep shows multinucleate giant cells Distinguish from HSV by culture or FA stain
Kaposi's Sarcoma (KS)	Firm subcutaneous brown-black or purple nodules, any cutaneous site esp. face, chest, genitals, extremities	Must distinguish from bacillary angiomatosis Biopsy
Molluscum contagiosum	Pearly white or flesh colored papules with central umbilication; most common on face and genitals	Usually clinical appearance EM of scraping of vesicle fluid
Psoriasis	Plaques that are sharply demarcated, esp knees, elbows, scalp, lumbosacral area	Biopsy with histopath may resemble seborrhea or drug eruption
Seborrhea	Erythematous, scaling plaques with indistinct margins, esp scalp, butterfly region of face, ears, hairline, chest, upper back, axilla, groin	Clinical features
Staph aureus	Folliculitis ± pruritis, esp trunk, groin, face	Exudate should show typical GPC and grow S. aureus

INDEX

Note: Page numbers in *italics* refer to figures; page numbers followed by t refer to tables.